APPLICATIONS MANUAL

APPLICATIONS MANUAL

to accompany DATA
ANALYSIS &
STATISTICS
FOR NURSING RESEARCH

Denise F. Polit, PhD
Humanalysis, Inc.
Saratoga Springs, New York

Appleton & Lange
Stamford, Connecticut

96 97 98 99 00 / 10 9 8 7 6 5 4 3 2 1

Prentice Hall International (UK) Limited, *London*
Prentice Hall of Australia Pty. Limited, *Sydney*
Prentice Hall Canada, Inc., *Toronto*
Prentice Hall Hispanoamericana, S.A., *Mexico*
Prentice Hall of India Private Limited, *New Delhi*
Prentice Hall of Japan, Inc., *Tokyo*
Simon & Schuster Asia Pte. Ltd., *Singapore*
Editora Prentice Hall do Brasil Ltda., *Rio de Janeiro*
Prentice Hall, *Upper Saddle River, New Jersey*

ISBN   0-8385-6334-1

Acquisitions Editor: David P. Carroll
Editor-in-Chief, Nursing: Sally J. Barhydt
Production: Andover Publishing Services
Designer: Libby Schmitz

9 780838 563342

90000

PRINTED IN THE UNITED STATES OF AMERICA

Contents

Preface

This Applications Manual was designed to accompany the textbook *Data Analysis and Statistics for Nursing Research*—although students using a different basic statistics text also could benefit from using it. The primary goal of this manual is to provide opportunities for hands-on computer experience with data analysis. The manual includes a large data set on a diskette at the back of the book and statistical exercises arranged in chapters corresponding to each chapter in the textbook. (We note, however, that some of the exercises can be done without the use of the computer; one-third of the exercises in each chapter are designed to help students read and interpret computer printouts of statistical analyses that have already been performed and that are reproduced here.)

The manual does not provide instructions on how to use a computer, nor on how to use any specific statistical software package. We assume that instructors or computer center personnel will be available to assist students with basic set-ups (or to *do* the actual installation of the computer files, and then provide students with specific instructions on how to access the files on personal computers designated for the analyses).

Students will need to carefully read Part I of this manual before proceeding with the exercises in Part II. However, we suggest that they review Chapter 1 in the textbook before delving into Part I of this manual. Students will be better prepared to learn about the data set if they understand some basic terms, such as **variable** and **data**.

We hope that users of this manual will profit from the opportunity to explore a rich and varied data set using their developing statistical skills.

Denise F. Polit

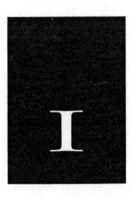

Introduction to the Applications Manual

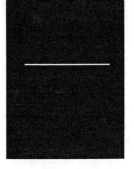

Introduction

A. RATIONALE FOR THE APPLICATIONS MANUAL

This Applications Manual was developed based on a conviction that the best way to learn about data analysis is to *do* it, not just read about it. Statistical analyses are now almost always performed on a computer, often on a personal computer. With the widespread availability of personal computers and appropriate statistical software, it is now practical—if not imperative—to perform computerized statistical analyses as part of a course on basic statistics.

We have prepared exercises for this Applications Manual that are designed to give you realistic data analytic experiences with a large data set. The exercises have been crafted to reinforce the material covered in the accompanying textbook on a chapter-by-chapter basis.

The purpose of this manual, then, is to promote active learning of statistics and data analysis. An attractive feature is that we have included a *real* data set—data that come from a very large, longitudinal study that began in 1979 and that is still ongoing. Thus, the analyses you undertake will have a real-world feel to them. As you work through the exercises, you will be testing realistic and interesting hypotheses and answering provocative questions using real data from a large survey sample.

It must be acknowledged that we faced a challenge in preparing this manual. Computer software and hardware are constantly being revised and created, and even as we go to press we risk the danger of making statements that will soon be outdated. Moreover, there are already numerous different computers, operating systems, and statistical software packages that could be used to analyze data—too many for us to provide detailed instructions for installing the data file on any given computer. Therefore, **we do not give step-by-step instructions in this manual on how to operate a personal computer, nor on how to access a statistical software package, nor on how to install the diskette that is enclosed with this manual.** We do provide some detailed examples that we believe will accommodate a large number of users of the manual, but in most cases it will be essential for you to have access to a person who can assist with the basic set-up of the computer files before you can proceed with the analyses. That person will often be the instructor teaching the statistics course, but in other cases will be an assistant at a computer facility.

As you proceed through this book, you will be exposed to the challenges and rewards of a researcher/analyst. Hundreds—even thousands—of analytic possibilities lie before you. It is a great adventure, and one that we hope will ignite your curiosity as you gain important new skills.

B. OVERVIEW OF WHAT IS INCLUDED

The Applications Manual consists of this printed manual and a 3½-inch diskette with several computer files. Here follows an overview of these two components and a discussion of what is *not* included with the manual.

1. The Manual

The manual has three main parts. Part I is designed to provide you with the necessary background for undertaking computer analyses with a real data set. In this introductory section we discuss the key features of the data set, the variables that are in the data set, the technical requirements for analyzing the data, software options, and other important issues relating to the use of the data set.

Part II of the manual consists of 14 chapters, each corresponding to a chapter in the textbook. Each chapter, in turn, contains three types of exercises. The first type is called "Directed Computer Exercises," which are specific analytic exercises to be performed using the data set on the diskette. Each exercise is followed by a series of questions, which require you to examine and interpret the printouts resulting from the computer analyses. The answers to these questions are included in Appendix D to facilitate learning and to ensure that you have a second opportunity to perform the appropriate analyses. The second type of exercise is called "Independent Computer Exercises." Here, you are encouraged to develop and test your own hypotheses using data from the diskette. Specific suggestions for analyses that could be performed are offered. The third type of exercise is called "Exercises in Reading Computer Printouts." These exercises include several computer printouts that you must digest and interpret in order to address the accompanying questions. The printouts are based on the analysis of another large-scale data set with over 2000 cases. Thus, these exercises do not require you to perform analyses, but they *do* require you to be able to comprehend computer printouts of statistical analyses. The answers to the questions for these exercises also are included at the back of the book.

Part III of the manual is the appendix section. Most of the appendixes (Appendixes A to C) offer information on the data set—what the variables are, how missing values are treated, what the codes mean, and so on. The final appendix (Appendix D) provides answers to most questions in Part II.

2. The Diskette

The diskette (located in the sleeve of the manual's back cover) contains three computer files (we say more about *files* in a subsequent section of Part I). One file (named NLSY.DAT) consists of the actual data available for analysis. These data are from a sample of nearly 1500 women and their first-born children. Over 100 variables, most of which are health-related, are included in the file, providing ample opportunity to address interesting research questions. We describe the data at greater length in a subsequent section of this introduction.

Because the first file on the diskette contains raw data (that is, the actual numerical values for all variables), it is possible for you to use *any* statistical software package you wish for performing the statistical analyses—on any type of personal computer that can handle statistical software. By using the information in Appendix A, you could create software-specific statements to communicate to the computer such information as the variable names and variable locations in conjunction with the data file. However, generating the statements to read raw data is a laborious process. Therefore, as a convenience to many of you, we decided to include the relevant commands for two of the most widely used statistical software packages—SPSS/PC and SAS/PC.[1] In both cases, the commands on the diskette are for current versions of the software as used on an IBM-compatible computer with the operating system known as MS-DOS (Microsoft Disk Operating System). Modifications to the commands in these two files would be needed for use with different computers (e.g., SPSS/Mac for Apple Macintosh computers) or with different operating systems (e.g., OS/2, or Operating System/2).

SPSS/PC (which on your system may be referred to as SPSS/PC+) is the personal computer version of the Statistical Package for the Social Sciences. SPSS is perhaps the most popular software package available for learning about basic statistical analysis. The commands for using SPSS are relatively simple, and no prior experience with statistical software is necessary (although familiarity with a computer keyboard and basic computer operations is assumed). Versions of SPSS have been available for mainframe

---

[1]Throughout this manual and the accompanying text, trademarked names (such as SPSS) are used. Rather than using a trademark symbol for each occurrence of such trademarked names, we formally note here that we are using the names in a purely editorial and pedagogical fashion, to the benefit of the trademark owner, with no intention of infringement upon the trademark.

computers and personal computers for over 25 years, and thus we expect that many instructors will be familiar with SPSS. All of the computer examples in the textbook were produced by SPSS/PC+ (we generally will refer to the software henceforth as SPSS, rather than SPSS/PC or SPSS/PC+, for simplicity). Moreover, throughout this manual we offer "SPSS Tips," specific guidance on how to perform the analyses suggested in the directed computer exercises. There is no question that those of you who are using SPSS will find this manual especially user-friendly. The SPSS commands for using the NLSY data set are in the file named NLSY.SPS.

SAS/PC is the personal computer version of the software package known as the Statistical Analysis System. SAS is generally considered to be somewhat more sophisticated, from a statistical point of view, than SPSS. The syntax of SAS is fairly easy to learn, and SAS for personal computers is also widely available. The SAS/PC commands for using the NLSY data set are in the file labeled NLSY.SAS.

3. What Is Not Included with the Manual

This manual does not include the statistical software needed to perform data analysis. A wide variety of statistical software exists for IBM compatible and Apple Macintosh computers, including SPSS, SAS, BMD-P, Crunch, and many others. Since the manual includes a raw data file, it should be possible to use any statistical software package to perform the exercises in this book, but the process admittedly will be easier for those using SAS and, especially, SPSS.

The manual assumes basic familiarity with the computer—with the keyboard, function keys, the mouse (if applicable), the monitor, etc. As noted earlier, the manual does not provide step-by-step instructions for installing and using the files because there are too many different computers, operating systems, environments (windows or no windows), software packages, menu systems, and editors to make such specificity feasible. Therefore, we assume that you are either sufficiently familiar with the basic functioning of the computer you will be using to install the files *or* that you have available to you someone who has this knowledge and can help you. In the final section of Part I, we *do* provide an example of a step-by-step installation process that is likely to be helpful to many of you.

C. THE NLSY DATA SET

The National Longitudinal Survey of Labor Market Experiences of Youth (NLSY) is an ongoing study that was initiated in 1979. The original purpose of the survey was to collect information on the employment-related characteristics and experiences of a cohort of young people. However, over the years the scope of the survey has broadened and diversified, and the survey now collects data annually from the same panel of respondents on health, marriage and fertility, emotional well-being, child rearing and child care, and many other important topics. Thousands of research reports, journal articles, theses, and dissertations have been based on NLSY data. The data included on the diskette with this Applications Manual are an extract (a subset of cases and variables) from the NLSY data set.

1. The NLSY Sample

The original sample for the NLSY survey was a national probability sample of 5831 young women and 5575 young men who, at the time of the initial interview in 1979, were between the ages of 14 and 21. The sampling method used (multistage, stratified random sampling) was designed to yield a database that could be statistically projected to represent the entire noninstitutionalized population born between 1957 and 1964 in the United States, as well as substantively important subgroups within this population. The sample includes an overrepresentation of Hispanics, African-Americans, and economically disadvantaged whites, so that meaningful analyses of separate racial/ethnic and socioeconomic groups could be conducted.

The NLSY sample has been reinterviewed annually since 1979—mostly in face-to-face interviews conducted in the respondents' homes. Rates of attrition (dropping out of the study) have been very low, with a completion rate of about 92% of the original sample through 1986—the year the data on the enclosed diskette are from, for the most part.

2. The Mother-Child Sample

The 1986 survey of the NLSY included a special supplement consisting of an extensive battery of assessment information for all children of the female NLSY respondents. Assessments were completed with a total of 4971 children, about 95% of those who were eligible. These children were born to approximately 3000 women from the original NLSY sample who had become mothers by 1986. The assessments included measures of the cognitive, socioemotional, and health aspects of each child's development, as well as information about the quality of parenting and the home environment. Some information about the children was provided by the mothers, but most assessment materials were administered directly to the children. These children continue to be part of the NLSY study and are reassessed every two years. (Infants born to the NLSY women between assessment waves are added to the sample.)

3. The NLSY Extract File

The data set included with this Applications Manual is an extract from the 1986 merged mother-child file.[2] The extract file includes a total of 138 variables (i.e., responses to interview questions or scales) for a subsample of 1455 mother-child cases. In selecting cases and variables from the larger data set, two competing considerations had to be bal-

---

[2] The full merged mother-child file for 1986 contains data on several thousand variables for 4971 children; a mainframe computer is typically required to analyze this enormous data set.

anced—first, the need to have a data set that was small enough to be stored on a diskette, and second, the desire to have an interesting and varied data set with a sufficiently large number of cases to permit analyses of subgroups (for example, analyses focusing on Hispanic children).

The Extract Subsample.   To ensure a sample of manageable size, only one child per family was selected for the extract data set. In the extract file, the focal child (referred to throughout as the Child) is the first-born child of an NLSY mother. The sample was further constrained by retaining only focal Children who were younger than 6 years of age at the time of the 1986 interview. Cases with extensive amounts of missing data for the variables in the data set were also deleted. It is important to recognize that, because of the constraints placed on the selection of cases, *the sample cannot be considered representative of all NLSY children, nor of the population of children born to American women who were aged 21 to 28 in 1986.*[3] The sample is intended to provide data analytic experiences, not to permit definitive inferences about a cohort of American preschoolers. Nevertheless, the sample is large and diverse with regard to geographic, racial/ethnic, and socioeconomic representation.

The Extract Variables.   The data set includes a broad range of variables about the focal Child and his or her mother. Most of the variables are from the 1986 NLSY survey, but information about the mother was drawn from interviews dating back to the original 1979 interview. The variables, most of which are health-related, are described at greater length in a subsequent section.

D. COMPUTER FILES

Before describing the variables in the NLSY extract file, we need to review some terminology that will be useful in working with the data. The terminology focuses on various **files** that are used in processing the data and performing analyses.[4]

Most computer files can be named and used over and over again. Computer files can be stored on the computer's hard disk or, if sufficiently small, on a diskette. File names are usually from one to eight characters in length, with an extension of up to three characters that must be separated from the main name by a period. Examples include FILEA.DAT and NLSYFILE.INC. File names must begin with an alphabetical character, but can contain numbers, as in FILE1.DAT. Blanks within the file name (e.g., FILE 1.DAT) are *not* allowed.

---

[3]Weighting is sometimes used to derive population estimates when stratified probability samples have been drawn. The original NLSY sample was a stratified, multistage sample, and there are weights associated with each case in the merged mother-child file. However, these weights would not have been appropriate for the extract data set, given the unusual selection criteria used to reduce the size of the sample for student use.

[4]There are other types of files that are not discussed here (e.g., portable files, results files, log files, etc.). The manual for the software package you are using can be consulted for a description of other files.

1. Data File

A **data file** contains the raw data values from a study. In a survey, the data values are the numbers or codes corresponding to people's responses to questions they've been asked in the interviews.

- **The file NLSY.DAT on the enclosed diskette is the name of the data file containing the NLSY extract data.**

Box 1 shows a very small portion of the NLSY.DAT file—the data for five cases (that is, for five mothers and their first-born children).

The numbers in a raw data file are arranged in rows and columns. In the NLSY.DAT file, the data for each case require 7 rows, arranged in 80 columns. Within each case, a row is called a **record.** The last column in each row (column 80) specifies the record number within a case. Thus, column 80 always contains a record number from 1 to 7, in consecutive order within the case.

The first four columns in each record contain the identification (ID) number for the case. Thus, we can see in Box 1 that the ID number for the first case (rows 1 through 7) is 1001 and the ID number for the second case (rows 8 through 14) is 1004. Thus, altogether the data file on the diskette consists of 10,185 rows of numerical data (7 records per case × 1455 cases).

The remaining numbers are the data values for the variables in the file. The numbers are arranged in **fixed format,** which means that specific columns in a given row always correspond to the same variable for all cases. For example, on record 1, columns 6 and 7 are used to store information on the month in which the 1986 interview was conducted for each case. We can see in Box 1 that the mother-child pair with ID number 1001 was interviewed in month 3 (March), while the mother-child pair with ID number 1004 was interviewed in month 5 (May). The data in the file were formatted to have blanks between each variable. Thus, for each case, column 5 is always blank because the ID number is separated from the next adjacent variable by a blank. Appendix A indicates the row and column location of every variable on the NLSY.DAT file.

2. Program File

To access, manipulate, and analyze the data, the computer must be told what each variable in the data file represents. For example, the computer must be told that columns 1 through 4 represent an ID number, just as we needed to communicate that information to you in this manual. A **program file** describes the variable names and locations and tells the computer what the codes mean.[5]

A program file is specific to the software being used to analyze the data. Thus, while the NLSY.DAT file will be used by everyone using the Applications Manual, dif-

---

[5]For small data sets, the data can be entered directly into the program file without having a separate data file. However, this would not be practical for large data sets such as the NLSY.

BOX 1

DATA FOR FIVE CASES IN THE NLSY EXTRACT FILE

```
1001   3 86   3   2   6 81 56   4 -1 28   4  1  1  0  1  0  0  0  0  0  8 61 24 19   1
1001   770   2 10 80 98 98   0     0  30000   0  4 -1   6 100  2 10 16 10 14   0   2
1001   0 32   7 21   3   2   7   3   4 118 113 114   -1  99  89 102  83  99 119 120   3
1001   2 -1 -1  93 102   -1  -1  -1  97  1 -1 10  1  0  1  1  1  1  1  0  0   4
1001   0  32  32   5  1  0  0  0  3  7  1  0  0  0 42 36  1  0  1 12  1 13  1   5
1001  18  0 -1  0 -1  0 -1  1 18  1  2  1  0  3  0  1  0  1  1  1  4 126 70 40   6
1001   1 162 21   8   8                                                              7
1004   5 86   3   1 12 82 41   3 -1   0   4   0  1  0  1  1  0  1  1  1 11 58 27 24   1
1004  460   2   8 81 98 98   0     0    -1  0  1 30   0   0  3 13 19 12 16   0   2
1004   0 35   7 19   3   2   9   4   4  97       87 107  -1  -1  -1  -1  -1  -1  -1   3
1004  -1 -1 -1  -1  -1  -1  -1  -1  -1  1 14  2  1  1  0  1  1  1  1  1  12   4
1004  12 20  20  20   0   0   0  1  2  7  1  0  0  0 -1 42  0 -1 -1  0 -1  0   5
1004  -1  0 -1  0 -1  0 -1  0 -1  1  1  1  4  0  1  1  0  1  0  1  1 150 42 39   6
1004   0 104 20   3   4                                                              7
1005   3 86   3   2 10 82 40   3 -1   0   5   0  0  2  0  1  0  0  1  1  6 61 24 21   1
1005  395   1 99 99 99 99   0     0    -1  1  1 40  14  55  3 15 17 12 12   0   2
1005   0      9 14   2  1  0  2  2 77 94 64 119  -1  -1  -1  -1  -1  -1 -1   3
1005   2 -1 10 108  90   -1  -1  -1  81  1 -1  3  1  0  1  1  1  1  0  0   4
1005   0 22  22  12   0   0   0  2  2  7  1  0  0  0 38 30  1 16  1 11  1 16  0   5
1005  -1  0 -1  0 -1  0 -1  0 -1  1  4  0  1  2  0  1  0  1  0  0  1 125 55 39   6
1005   0 98 19   4   4                                                               7
1006   3 86   3   2   9 81 53   4 -1 46   4  1  1  0  1  0  0  0  0  0  4 61 24 20   1
1006  710   2 11 80 98 98   0     0  28000   0  4 -1   3 73  0 11 19 12 14   0   2
1006   0 34 13 16   3   4   3   4   4 114 119  98  -1 101  89 122 106 108  87  97   3
1006   1 -1 -1 100 102   -1  -1  -1 112  1 -1 12  1  0  1  1  1  1  1  0  0   4
1006   0 36  45  16   0   0   1  1  3  2  1  0  0  0 40 34  1 18  1 14  0 -1  0   5
1006  -1  0 -1  0 -1  0 -1  1  1  1  0  0  0  1  0  1  0  4  4 100 18 39   6
1006   0 103 19   3   3                                                              7
1007   4 86   3   1 12 82 39   3 -1   0   3   0  1  0  1  0  0  1  1  1  5 58 27 24   1
1007  930   2   6 78 98 98   0     0  40908   0  1 35   0   0  3 12 19 14 16   0   2
1007   0 38 11 12   3   5   7   3   3 115 120 102  98  -1  -1  -1  -1  -1  -1  -1   3
1007   4 -1 10  83  90   -1  -1  -1 117  1 -1  1  2  0  1  1  1  1  1  1  16   4
1007  10 48  48   8   0   0   0  1  2  1  1  0  0  0 36 35  1 18  1 10  1 18  0   5
1007  -1  0 -1  0 -1  0 -1  1  2  1  3  0  0  1  0  1  0  4  1 145 41 41   6
1007   0 139 21   5   5                                                              7
```

ferent students will need different program files. We have included on the diskette two program files:

- **NLSY.SPS is the name of the program file for those using SPSS/PC on an IBM-compatible computer using MS-DOS.**
- **NLSY.SAS is the name of the program file for those using SAS/PC on an IBM-compatible computer using MS-DOS.**

For those using a statistical software package other than SPSS and SAS, a program file will need to be created, using information in Appendixes A and C. For those using SPSS or SAS in a different environment (e.g., on Apple Macintosh computers or with the OS/2 Operating System), modifications to the program files will be necessary.

Each of the two program files on the diskette contains instructions to the computer with regard to the following:

- *Variable name*   The name of each variable, as it must be used in subsequent analyses
- *Variable location*   The record and column location for each variable
- *Variable label*   A label that describes what each variable is; the label is longer than the variable name and therefore is more informative
- *Value label*   A label describing each numeric value, when that value is not self-evident (e.g. if the value for the Child's gender is 1, the label indicates that the Child is male; however no label is used for a variable like family income because the value is a straightforward dollar amount).
- *Missing values*   The value that is used when a case has no information for a variable, i.e., the code used when a respondent did not answer (or was not asked) a question.

The SPSS and SAS program files should be directly usable for reading the NLSY.DAT file for most of you with IBM-compatible personal computers with MS-DOS.

3. Command File

Instructions for performing specific analyses can be stored in a **command file.**[6] For example, if we wanted the computer to calculate what percentage of the sample was male and female, we could enter the necessary commands into a command file and then instruct the computer to execute that file.

Command files need not be named and saved if you are working in an **interactive mode.** If you work interactively, commands can be typed onto the keyboard one at a time and submitted for processing, and then the results can be reviewed before typing the next command. The interactive mode is particularly convenient for running simple analyses that you want performed immediately. However, one advantage of working with named command files is that they can be saved and then edited for further analyses. For example, if we wanted to compute the average age of the focal Children, and then the next day realized we also wanted to compute the average age of the mothers, the original command could be easily edited by retrieving the command file and replacing one variable name for the other, rather than starting a new file and retyping the entire command. For complex analyses, this is very attractive.

Commands for any desired analyses could also be placed at the end of the program file. However, it is cumbersome to redefine the variables with the program file every time an analysis is performed. Command files used with systems files (described next) are the most efficient method of performing analyses.

---

[6]Some authors make no distinction between a command file and a program file, because both are used to communicate commands to the computer in the syntax specific to the software.

4. Systems File

A **systems file** (referred to in SAS as a **SAS dataset**) merges a data file with a program file, so that variables do not have to be defined on each computer run. The systems file contains all of the raw data, together with information on variable names, variable locations, variable labels, value labels, and missing values codes. By using a systems file, the desired analysis can be processed immediately and requires much less time to run. This is particularly advantageous for a large data set like the NLSY.

- **For users of SPSS or SAS, the program file has been preprogrammed to create a systems file (SAS dataset) that will be stored on your hard disk.**

That is, the program file on the diskette contains the command to create a systems file, which can be used in all subsequent analyses in lieu of the program file.

Users of SPSS create and save a systems file through the "SAVE OUTFILE" command at the end of the program file. The systems file will be stored in the same directory on your hard disk as the one used to store your software package.[7]

- **NLSY.SYS is the name of the systems file that will be created by those using SPSS after executing the program file NLSY.SPS.**

Users of SAS save a permanent SAS dataset by defining a LIBNAME and using it in the DATA statement that precedes the listing of variabl names and position numbers. The SAS dataset created by NLSY.SAS will be stored in the NLSY directory on your hard disk.

- **NLSY.SSD is the name of the SAS dataset that will be created by those using SAS after executing NLSY.SAS.**

After creating the systems file (or SAS dataset), you need only enter commands to access that file and instruct the computer to perform the desired analyses. For example, suppose we wanted to compute the average age in months of the focal Children in the NLSY sample, using SPSS. We could create a small command file with the following instructions:

GET FILE = 'NLSYS.SYS'.
DESCRIPTIVES VARIABLES=BCAGEMON.

The first command tells the computer to retrieve the systems file, which is named NLSYS.SYS. The second command is the SPSS-specific instruction to compute several descriptive statistics, including averages, for the variable in the systems file named BCAGEMON (the focal Child's age in months at the time of the 1986 interview). By

---

[7]For those not wishing to create a systems file, the commands can be deleted from the program file using an editor. We strongly recommend, however, that a systems file (SAS dataset) be created.

executing the command file, the desired analysis would be performed. (In SAS, a comparable analysis could be performed with a PROC MEANS statement, following the definition of the LIBNAME.)

5. Active File

The file used in an analytic session is called the **active file** (or, in SAS, a **temporary file**). An active file is created internally in the computer during the course of performing an analytic operation. An active file is created by executing a program file or command file with a raw data file or a systems file. Active files are not named or saved, and are generally "invisible" to the analyst.

6. Listing File

The results of an analysis can be displayed directly on the computer monitor. However, it is often desirable to print the results from a listing file that can later be printed. A **listing file** contains a copy of the results generated by executing a command file. In SPSS, results from a run are stored in the listing file named SPSS.LIS.[8] SAS automatically saves a listing file that has the same name as the program being executed, but with a .LST extension. The listing file can be printed whenever it is convenient to do so. The listing file is maintained on the computer's hard drive until a specific command is made to delete it (or until it is overwritten by another run).

7. Log File

A **log file** contains the commands that the software program has executed during a session, in the order the commands were submitted and executed. In addition, the log file contains feedback from the program with respect to the commands. For example, the log file includes error messages about commands that could not be executed, warnings (problems encountered that did not prevent execution of the commands), and other notes. The log file can be reviewed on the monitor or printed. In SPSS, the log file for a session is named SPSS. LOG. In SAS, the log file has the same name as the program being executed, but with a .LOG extension.

E. VARIABLES IN THE NLSY EXTRACT DATA SET

To use the NLSY data set in the exercises described in Part II of this Applications Manual, you must be familiar with the variables. As noted earlier, there are 138 variables in the file, and these variables can be used to perform hundreds of different analyses. This section provides an overview of the variables available for analysis.

---

[8]Because the SPSS.LIS file is automatically overwritten by any subsequent run, it is often desirable to create a separate listing file for each computer run with a user-defined name, through a SET LIST command.

1. Variable Topics

The variables in the NLSY.DAT file have been clustered into eight main topic areas. These topic areas, with the associated two-letter prefix used in naming the variables, are as follows:

- *Administrative (AD) Variables.* Administrative variables, such as a case identification number
- *Background of the Child (BC) Variables.* Variables that are primarily demographic in nature, indicating background characteristics of the focal Child (e.g., the Child's gender)
- *Background of the Mother (BM) Variables.* Variables that are primarily demographic in nature, indicating background characteristics of the mother (e.g., the mother's age)
- *Child Development (CD) Variables.* Variables from the cognitive and psychosocial assessments of the focal Child (e.g., scores on the Behavior Problem Index)
- *Child Health (HL) Variables.* Indicators of the Child's physical and health status (e.g., the Child's weight)
- *Maternal Drug Use (MD) Variables.* Mother's use of various drugs and her age at first use (e.g., the age when she first tried marijuana)
- *Pregnancy/Childbirth (PR) Variables.* Variables concerning the mother's pregnancy with and delivery of the focal Child (e.g., whether the mother received prenatal care)

2. Variable Names

All the variables in the NLSY data set have been assigned names. The names comply with the rules for variable naming in most statistical software packages—that is, the names all begin with an alphabetic character and contain no more than eight characters.

Certain conventions have been adopted in naming the variables to help you use the variables conveniently:

- *First two letters.* The first two letters indicate the broad topic area of the variable. The listing of the topic areas in the previous section indicates the two letters used, in parentheses. For example, variables beginning with BM are always background of the mother variables.
- *Middle letters.* After the first two letters, the variable name tries to capture the essence of the variable, insofar as possible within the eight-character constraint. For example, BCRACE is a background of the Child variable (BC) that indicates the Child's race/ethnicity.
- *Date Information.* The last two digits of the variable name are sometimes used to indicate the survey year in which the information was obtained. For example, the variable BMSE80 is a background of the mother variable (BM) measuring self-esteem (SE) on a scale that was administered in the 1980 interview (80).

For the most part, *variables that do not end with a two-digit number were measured in the 1986 interview.* For example, the variable BMHIGRAD indicates the mother's highest grade of education completed at the time of the 1986 interview. The year 1986 is implied by the absence of any numbers at the end of the variable name.

However, other variables without the two-digit numerical suffix omit the survey year for other reasons. First, some variables inherently convey time-related information. For example, the variable BMAGEMEN is a variable indicating the mother's age at menarche. The year in which that variable was measured is not important, since the variable itself is age-specific. A more common reason for omitting the year-of-measurement information in the variable name is that some variables were measured in different survey years for different women, depending on when the focal Child was born. For example, the focal Child's birth weight was measured in the survey year following his or her birth. Since the Children range in age from newborns to 5-year-olds, birth weight information was gathered at some point between 1980 to 1986. In general, then, **the year-of-interview information is included as part of the variable name when it is important to know that the variable captures a transient status for some point prior to 1986.** For example, the mother's self-esteem in 1980 is not necessarily the same as self-esteem in 1986, but her age at menarche and the Child's birth weight would be the same (except for recall problems) no matter when the question was asked.

Although we have tried to use variable names that imply the meaning of the variable, eight characters are rarely adequate for conveying what the underlying concept is. The program files include extended variable labels that communicate more clearly than the variable names what was being measured. When analyses are performed, these variable labels generally appear on the printouts so that the statistical results are more intelligible.

3. Variable Codes

All of the data in the NLSY data set are numeric. Some of the variables are inherently quantitative (e.g., the Child's height in inches) and these numbers are the values that appear in the file. Most variables, however, have been coded, and the meaning of the codes is not obvious. Appendixes B and C of this Applications Manual provide information on how the NLSY variables were coded.

Most of the dichotomous variables (variables with only two response options, such as yes or no) use the codes of 1 or 0. For these variables, it is often possible to infer the codes directly through the variable name. For example, the variable PRCARE (whether the mother received prenatal care when she was pregnant with the focal Child) is coded 1 if the mother did receive prenatal care and 0 if she did not.

The program files include labels for all coded values. As with variable labels, these value labels appear on printouts of requested analyses to facilitate interpretation of the results.

4. Missing Values

In a survey, it is rare for all respondents to answer every question on the interview schedule. Sometimes a respondent refuses to answer a question, and sometimes an interviewer forgets to ask a question. Most missing values occur, however, because of legitimate skip patterns. For example, if question 1 asks if the respondent has been hospitalized in the past 12 months and question 2 asks the reason for the hospitalization, those who answered "no" to question 1 would skip over question 2. Thus, missing values are common in survey-based data sets.

When data are missing, codes are assigned to the relevant variables to indicate the absence of valid information. Prior to running an analysis, it is imperative to communicate to the computer what the missing values codes are. In the NLSY data set, **the missing values code for all variables is –1.** An inspection of Box 1 shows that the five first cases in the file have a number of variables coded -1. In the program files created for users of SAS and SPSS, the missing values codes have already been specified. For most analyses, the cases with missing values on the variables in the analysis are simply omitted. For example, if 10 out of 100 respondents failed to indicate their age, the computer would compute the average age based on 90 cases, not 100.

It is important to note that in some analyses, you will need to declare additional missing values. For example, in the NLSY data set the variable BMHIGRAD (mother's highest grade completed) has codes indicating the number of years of schooling, ranging from 0 (no formal schooling) to 18 (6+ years of college). However, there is an additional code of 95 for those who attended school in an ungraded program. The cases with the code of 95 would have to be omitted (or perhaps recoded) if you wanted to compute the mothers' average educational attainment, because the code 95 does not represent 95 years of education. Thus, it is important to refer to the codebook (Appendix B or C) whenever variables are being used in an analysis.

5. Using Appendixes A, B and C

The first three appendixes at the end of this Applications Manual are the keys to the variable names and codes. Each appendix serves a somewhat different purpose.

- *Appendix A* lists the 138 variables in the order they appear in the NLSY.DAT file. The only information in this appendix is variable name, variable location (i.e., what record and column the data are in), format (width of the field, i.e., the number of columns allocated), and variable label. Information in this appendix is critical to those who need to create a program file to use the NLSY data with a software package other than SAS or SPSS.
- *Appendix B* provides more detailed information on the meaning of the variables. For many variables, this appendix specifies the exact wording of the question as asked in the interviews and the response alternatives. For variables that represent the scores on scales created by combining responses to multiple questions, an explanation of the scoring and examples of the items are provided. Appendix B lists variables in the order they appear in the NLSY.DAT file.
- *Appendix C* is computer-generated codebook for all variables in the file, listed *in alphabetical order.* This appendix specifies the variable names and labels, the codes and code labels, and the missing values.

F. VARIABLE CREATION

The analyses that can be performed with the NLSY data set are not limited to the 138 variables as they are constructed on the enclosed disk. You can manipulate the data to create new variables, and all statistical software packages offer many types of commands for variable creation. We will give you some examples of variable creation so that you can be alert to various opportunities for enhancing the analytic potential of the NLSY data.

1. *Conditional Variables.* Values from existing variables that meet a specific condition can be used as the basis for creating new variables. For example, the NLSY data set includes the variable BMAGE1ST, the age of the mother when she first gave birth. We could construct a new variable (named, for instance, TEENMOM) that contrasted mothers who had a baby while a teenager versus those who were 20 or older when they first gave birth. Such variables are typically created by using a series of "if then" statements. For example, if the code for BMAGE1ST is less than 20, then TEENMOM is coded 1, but if the code for BMAGE1ST is 20 or greater, then TEEN-MOM is coded 0.

2. *Recoded Variables.* Variables can often be changed simply by instructing the computer to recode values.[9] For example, the variable BMHIGRAD (years of education the mother completed) can be recoded such that values 11 and below are recoded to 0, and values 12 and above are coded to 1, thereby contrasting high school graduates with women who did not graduate from high school.

3. *Enumerated Variables.* It is sometimes useful to create a variable that is a count of values across other variables. For instance, the NLSY data set contains several variables relating to whether or not the mother ever used certain drugs (marijuana, amphetamines, barbiturates, cocaine, etc.). Each of these variables is coded 1 for women who ever used the drug and 0 otherwise. We could create for each case a new variable (e.g., DRUGNUM) that represented the number of different drugs the mother had ever used. DRUGNUM would be equal to the number of times a code of 1 occurred in the original drug use variables. Thus, if a woman had used only marijuana and nothing else, DRUGNUM would be set equal to 1; if another woman had used cocaine, psychedelics, and amphetamines, DRUGNUM would be set equal to 3.[10]

4. *Computed Variables.* Arithmetic operations can be used to create new variables through statistical software packages. For example, if we had responses to five questions, we might want to form a scale by adding the codes to the five questions together (e.g., SCALE = VAR1 + VAR2 + VAR3 + VAR4 + VAR5).

---

[9]Note that in SAS, there is no recode command, as there is in SPSS. Recoding must be done using if-then statements.
[10]In SPSS, enumerated variables can be created through the COUNT command. In SAS, counting must be done using a series of if statements, which can be streamlined through the use of arrays and iterative do loops.

Computed variables can involve simple mathematical operations like addition and subtraction, or can involve more complex transformations via mathematical **functions** that are available in statistical software packages (for example, rounding, truncating, raising the value to an exponential power, taking a square root, etc.). For example, the NLSY data set contains the variable PRBWT, the focal Child's birth weight in ounces. We might want to create another variable to indicate the Child's birth weight in pounds. In SPSS, we could use one of the following commands for a new variable we will call POUNDS:

COMPUTE   POUNDS = PRBWT/16.
COMPUTE   POUNDS = TRUNC (PRBWT/16).
COMPUTE   POUNDS = RND (PRBWT/16).

The first command would set the new variable POUNDS equal to the Child's birth weight in ounces (PRBWT), divided by 16—carried to two decimal places. The second command would set POUNDS equal to the infant's number of pounds at birth, truncating any fraction of a pound after the decimal place. Finally, the third command would set POUNDS equal to the infant's number of pounds at birth, rounded to the nearest whole number. As a concrete example, the value of PRBWT for the case with ID number 1004 (the second case in Box 1) is 104, which is 6.5 pounds. The computer would set POUNDS equal to 6.50 for the first command, 6 for the second command, and 7 for the third command. Of course, in a real analysis, only one of these commands would be used.

5. *Time-Related Variables.* The NLSY contains several variables that are dates (e.g., the month and year the mother first got married). These variables can be manipulated to yield interesting variables on duration (e.g., length of time first marriage lasted) or status at specific points in time (e.g., whether the mother was married when she first gave birth). Most software packages have a date function that can convert dates to the number of days elapsed since some specific point in time. In SPSS, for example, the YRMODA function sets a variable equal to the number of days elapsed since October 15, 1582, the first day of the Gregorian calendar. (The equivalent function in SAS is YMD.) Then these new date variables can be added, subtracted, or compared, to derive time-relevant variables such as duration.

The manual for the software you are using to analyze the NLSY data should be consulted to ascertain the commands needed to create new variables.

G. TECHNICAL REQUIREMENTS FOR USING THE DISKETTE

To use the accompanying diskette for data analysis, you will need to have access to a personal computer with a hard disk drive. The computer must have adequate memory for performing statistical analyses; a math coprocessor is recommended to speed up processing of the analyses.

To read the enclosed diskette, the computer must have a 3½ inch high-density floppy drive. Alternatively, if the computer you are using for statistical analysis has only a 5¼ inch high-density floppy drive, the files on the enclosed diskette can be copied onto a 5¼ inch diskette. To do this, you must have access to another computer that has both 5¼ inch and 3½ inch high-density drives.

The computer you are using to perform the statistical analyses must have a statistical software package installed on its hard drive. You must also have a manual that provides information on how to use the software package. (Although we provide users of SPSS many tips in this guidebook, these tips are not a substitute for the comprehensive advice and instructions offered in the SPSS manual.) Many statistical software packages, such as the personal computer version of SPSS, have a tutorial that is useful to go through before attempting actual analyses.

H. GETTING STARTED

As we noted earlier, it would not be possible for us to give step-by-step instructions for using the enclosed diskette that would be appropriate for all of you, given the many different types of hardware and software available. However, it is likely that many of you will be using either SPSS or SAS on an IBM-compatible computer that has an MS-DOS operating system, and so we provide in this section an example of a basic set-up for such situations. Even in these situations, it is likely that modifications to the commands shown in the example will be needed. We cannot know, for example, the name of the directory that contains your software system. We caution, then, that **the commands shown below are intended to be illustrative, not definitive.**

As we present commands in this section, we use the following conventions: material shown in all UPPER CASE are prompts from the computer; material shown in all lower case letters and bolded are commands that you need to type in; material shown in brackets { } are instructions for you to hit certain keys on the keyboard, such as {Enter}.

1. Setting up for SPSS

In this section, we provide an example of the installation of the program file and the data file for those using SPSS on an IBM-compatible computer using MS-DOS as the operating system. In this illustration, we assume that the program SPSSPC previously has been installed in the directory named SPSS on the C drive. It is possible that SPSSPC is located in a different directory on your machine, but the installation instructions for SPSSPC do suggest that the directory be named SPSS. If we were to install the NLSY program file for SPSS (NLSY.SPS) plus the NLSY data file (NLSY.DAT) *on our computer,* here are the steps we would need to take:

1) In the C drive, change the directory to SPSS, the directory where SPSSPC is stored, at the prompt:

C:\>cd spss{Enter}

2) Insert the diskette at the back of this manual into the drive for 3½ inch diskettes. (We assume that this is the A drive, but it could be the B drive; if it is B on your computer, substitute B for A in the following commands.)

3) Copy the data file from the diskette in drive A onto the C:\SPSS directory:

C:\SPSS>copy a:nlsy.dat{Enter}

The screen will show that one file has been copied.

4) Copy the SPSS program file from the diskette in drive A onto the C:\SPSS directory:

C:\SPSS>copy a:nlsy.sps{Enter}

The screen will show again that one file has been copied.

5) Remove the diskette from your A drive.

6) To run the program file, you will need to get into SPSS/PC, which requires a simple command:

C:\SPSS>spsspc{Enter}

7) When you start SPSS/PC you enter the Menu/Help System. You will see a screen with a menu on the upper left, a Help window on the upper right, and a "scratch pad" area in the lower half. The cursor light will be flashing in the upper left corner of the scratch pad. Once you are in the Menu/Help screen, hit the following function key:

{F10}

8) On the mini-menu that appears at the bottom of the screen, there are two commands shown after a prompt (RUN:)—Run from Cursor (highlighted) and Exit to Prompt. You want to exit to the prompt, so hit the right arrow cursor to highlight this command, and then execute the command by hitting the Enter key:

{Cursor right }{Enter}

You will then get a new prompt (SPSS/PC:) on the screen.

9) The next step is to execute the SPSS program file by typing in an include command. This will generate the systems file named NLSY.SYS:

SPSS/PC:inc 'nlsy.sps'.{Enter}

The commands in the SPSS program file will scroll up the screen as the program file is being executed. The screen will stop scrolling when it reaches a command that says SAVE OUTFILE='NLSY.SYS'. After several minutes, the computer will indicate that the procedure was completed (that the end of the include file has been reached), and the SPSS/PC: prompt will appear on the screen.

10) The systems file NLSY.SYS is now installed on the hard disk and can be accessed through a GET FILE instruction in a command file. (Command files can be built in the SPSS editor—called REVIEW—as described in the SPSS/PC manual. Command files can also be built in another editor/word processor[11] and then copied into the SPSS directory.) If no other operations are desired at this time, the session can be ended:

SPSS/PC:**finish.**{Enter}

11) This returns you to the C:\SPSS> prompt. If you wish, you can print a hard copy of the log file and listing file for confirmation that the program file was properly read and executed, and that a systems file was created:

C:\SPSS>**print spss.log**{Enter}
C:\SPSS>**print spss.lis**{Enter}

You could also print a hard copy of the NLSY.SPS commands, with the following command at the prompt:

C:\SPSS>**print nlsy.sps**{Enter}

12) When you have finished all printing, you can move into another directory with the change directory (cd) command.

2. Setting up for SAS

In this section, we provide an example of the installation of the program file and the data file for those using SAS on an IBM-compatible computer using MS-DOS as the operating system. These instructions can easily be adapted to any SAS platform, although they were created and tested in an MS-DOS environment.

1) On the C: drive, create a directory in which to store the data and program files:

C:\>**md nlsy**

2) Insert the diskette at the back of this manual into the drive for 3½-inch diskettes. (We assume that this is the A: drive, but it could be the B: drive; if it is B: on your computer, substitute B: for A: in the following commands.)

3) Copy the data file from the diskette in drive A: onto the C:\NLSY directory

C:\>**copy a:\nlsy.dat c:\nlsy**{Enter}

The screen will show that one file has been copied.

4) Now copy the SAS program file from the diskette in drive A: onto the C:\NLSY directory:

---

[11]If you are using a word processing program to build command files, it will almost certainly be necessary to convert the file to ASCII format—that is, to a text file that has been stripped of software-specific commands. Conversion to ASCII is typically a simple menu-driven routine. You should consult your word processing manual to determine how to perform such a conversion.

C:\>copy a:\nlsy.sas c:\nlsy{Enter}

The screen will again show that a file has been copied.

5) Remove the diskette from your A: drive.
6) Assuming that the SAS software is installed in the C:\SAS directory,[12] you can now run the program file by typing in the following commands:

C:\>cd nlsy
C:\NLSY>c:\sas\sas nlsy

7) SAS will execute the program NLSY.SAS and create the SAS dataset C:\NLSY\NLSY.SSD. The SAS dataset now can be accessed through a command file and used for analyses.
8) The execution of NLSY.SAS will create the log file C:\NLSY\NLSY.LOG and the list file C:\NLSY\NLSY.LST, both of which can be printed at the C:\NLSY> prompt if you wish to see the output:

C:\NLSY>print nlsy.log{Enter}
C\NLSY>print nlsy.lst{Enter}

You could also print a hard copy of the NLSY.SAS commands, with the following command at the prompt:

C:NLSY\>print nlsy.sas{Enter}

9) You will again be returned to the C:\NLSY> prompt. If there are no further analyses to be performed at this time, you can use the change directory (cd) command to move into another directory.

---

[12]If SAS is installed in another directory, simply substitute the directory for c:\sas in the instructions.

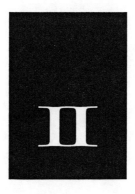

COMPUTER EXERCISES

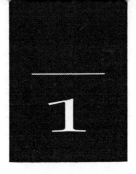

Introduction to Data Analysis

A. DIRECTED COMPUTER EXERCISES

Appendixes A, B, and C of this manual list all the variables in the NLSY data set contained on the enclosed diskette. (See Part I of this Manual for further information on the use of the data set and the accompanying files). Answer the following questions based on the NLSY data set.

    1. Focusing on variables that begin with **BC** (i.e., variables representing background characteristics of the focal Child) and using information in Appendix B or Appendix C, indicate which of the following variables are *discrete* and which are *continuous* (or capable of being continuous):

Variable Name	Continuous	Discrete
a. BCAGEMON	_____	_____
b. BCGRADE	_____	_____
c. BCHHSIZE	_____	_____
d. BCNSIBS	_____	_____
e. BCSPACNG	_____	_____

    2. Again focusing on **BC** (background of the Child) variables in the data set, indicate the level of measurement of each of the following variables:

Variable Name	Level of Measurement
a. BCRACE	_____
b. BCAGE	_____

c. BCFAINHH   _____

d. BCSPACNG   _____

e. BCSEEFA   _____

3. Review the **BM** variables—variables that are background characteristics of the mother. For each level of measurement (nominal, ordinal, interval, or ratio) identify one BM variable:

Nominal: _____

Ordinal: _____

Interval: _____

Ratio: _____

4. *Background.* Computer programs for statistical analysis generally have commands for displaying information about the variables in their file, such as what the variable names represent, what the valid codes are, how missing data are coded, and so on. Figure 1–1 illustrates such a display (from an SPSS-generated print-out) for the variables ADID and BCRACE in the NLSY data set.[1] (If a different software package were used, the display would naturally look somewhat different.)

For each specified variable, the computer prints the following information when the DISPLAY command is used with SPSS/PC:

Variable: Name of the variable in the file—eight digit maximum

Label: Variable label describing what the variable is—40 digit maximum

Value label: Label describing what individual codes mean—20 digit maximum for each label

Type: Indicator of whether the variable is numeric or alphabetic (string variable)

Width: Maximum number of columns allocated for the variable (i.e., maximum number of digits needed for all values of the variable)

Dec: Number of places to the right of the decimal point, if any

Missing: Code assigned to missing data

```
Variable: ADID           Label: CASE ID NUMBER
   No value labels       Type: Number  Width:  4  Dec: 0    Missing: * None *

Variable: BCRACE         Label: RACE-ETHNICITY OF CHILD
   Value labels follow   Type: Number  Width:  2  Dec: 0    Missing:   -1.00
      1.00   HISPANIC                              2.00   AFRICAN-AMERICAN
      3.00   NONHISP,NON AFR-AMERICAN
```

FIGURE 1–1. SPSS/PC PRINTOUT (DISPLAY) FOR VARIABLES ADID AND BCRACE

---

[1]Appendix C displays comparable information for *all* variables in the NLSY data set, listed in alphabetical order.

SPSS Tip[2]

The SPSS/PC command that created the printout in Figure 1–1 is:

DISPLAY ADID BCRACE.

DISPLAY is the command and ADID and BCRACE are the variables for which information is to be displayed.

In Figure 1–1, we see that the variable label for ADID is CASE ID NUMBER and that there are no value labels assigned to the codes for this variable. The variable ADID is a number that is 4 digits wide, with nothing to the right of the decimal point. There is no missing values code for ADID since all cases were assigned an identification number.

For the variable BCRACE (the *variable label* for which is RACE-ETHNICITY OF CHILD), the *missing* values code is −1. The *value labels* for actual codes are 1— HISPANIC, 2—AFRICAN-AMERICAN, and 3—NONHISP,NON AFR-AMERI-CAN. The maximum *width* of this *numeric* variable is 2; this accommodates the one digit needed for actual codes of 1, 2, or 3 and the two digits needed for the missing values code (−1). There are no places to the right of the *decimal place* for any code for BCRACE.

Exercise. Using the data files for the NLSY data set, display basic information for the following variables: BCGENDER, BCBIRTMO, BCBIRTYR, BCAGEMON, and BCAGE.[3]

When you have produced the display for the five specified variables, use the printout to answer the following questions:

a. Which variables use the code −1 for missing values?
b. Which variables have a width that is greater than 2?

---

[2]Throughout Part II we offer tips for those of you who are using SPSS to perform the statistical analyses. The tips use the syntax for SPSS/PC+, version 5.0 for MS-DOS. The commands might need to be modified slightly if you are using another version of SPSS.

[3]Different statistical software packages generate printouts that vary with regard to appearance and, in some instances, with regard to the information that is included as part of the program. Thus, **for those not using SPSS, it is possible that a few of the subquestions within the Directed Computer Exercises in this Manual cannot be answered** based on the printouts you will obtain.

SPSS Tip

In SPSS/PC, variables that are adjacent to one another in the file can be referenced with a TO command. For example, if we wanted to display ADID, ADINTMO, and ADINTYR—which are the first three consecutive variables in the NLSY file, as shown in Appendix A—we could use the following command:

DISPLAY ADID TO ADINTYR.

---

c. Which variables do not have any value labels for the codes?
d. If a focal Child was male, what code would be assigned to BCGENDER?
e. If a focal Child was 39 months old (BCAGEMON), would the value in BCAGE be 3.25 or 3?

   5. *Background.* Computer programs for statistical analysis generally have commands to list the *actual data values* for selected variables and selected cases. Such commands are often used in data cleaning or for preliminary inspection of the data. Figure 1–2 illustrates what an SPSS-generated listing looks like for the variables ADID to BCAGE (the first nine consecutive variables in the NLSY data set), for the first 10 cases in the file.
   The variable name for each of the nine variables is displayed in the top row of the listing. Beneath each variable is the *actual* data value for the first 10 cases in the file. For example, the first case has an identification number (ADID) of 1001. The interview for this case took place in March 1986 (ADINTMO = 3, ADINTYR = 86). The focal

ADID	ADINTMO	ADINTYR	BCRACE	BCGENDER	BCBIRTMO	BCBIRTYR	BCAGEMON	BCAGE
1001	3	86	3	2	6	81	56	4
1004	5	86	3	1	12	82	41	3
1005	3	86	3	2	10	82	40	3
1006	3	86	3	2	9	81	53	4
1007	4	86	3	1	12	82	39	3
1009	2	86	3	2	7	81	55	4
1011	2	86	3	1	11	82	39	3
1012	3	86	3	1	10	85	4	0
1013	4	86	3	2	10	80	65	5
1014	2	86	3	1	6	85	8	0

FIGURE 1–2. SPSS/PC PRINTOUT (LIST) FOR SELECTED VARIABLES AND CASES

SPSS Tip

The SPSS/PC command that created the printout in Figure 1–2 is:

LIST VARIABLES=ADID TO BCAGE
  /CASES=FROM 1 TO 10.

The SPSS program command is LIST, followed by the specification of which variables are to be listed. CASES= indicates that the listing should be done for the first 10 cases in the file (i.e., from case 1 to case 10).

Child is not Hispanic nor African-American (BCRACE = 3), is a female (BCGENDER = 2), and was born in June, 1981 (BCBIRTMO = 6, BCBIRTYR = 81). At the time of the 1986 interview, the Child was 56 months old (BCAGEMON = 56), which means that she was 4 years of age (BCAGE = 4). (Hint: When listing cases, it is always a good idea to list the identification number, along with the desired variables.)

Exercise. Using the data files for the NLSY data set, list the following variables for the first 10 cases: ADID, BCAGE, BC1STCC, BC2NDCC, and BC3RDCC. When you have produced the listing for the five specified variables, use the printout (and information on variable coding in Appendix C) to answer the following questions:

a. Of the first 10 cases in the NLSY file, how old is the youngest Child? How old is the oldest Child?
b. How many of the 10 Children in the listing used a regular child care arrangement during the first year of their lives?
c. What are the ID numbers of the four Children who used a regular child care arrangement in all *three* of the first years of their lives?
d. What is the ID number of the Child who first used a regular child care arrangement in the third year of his or her life?
e. What are the ID numbers of the two Children who have data missing for all three child care variables? Why are the data missing?

6. *Background.* When listing values of specific variables, as in Exercise A.5—or in performing many other analyses—it is often desirable to select a subset of the cases in the file. For example, we might want to list information on the variables ADID to

SPSS Tip

Several SPSS/PC commands could be used to select cases based on the Child's age, including the following:

SELECT IF (BCAGEMON LE 11).

PROCESS IF (BCAGEMON LE 11).

The first command (SELECT IF) could be used to select cases where the child's age (BCAGEMON) is less than or equal to (LE) 11 months *for all analyses being performed in the same computer run.* The second selection command (PROCESS IF) would apply *only to the command that follows immediately after,* which in this case is the LIST command. Various **relational operators** such as LE (less than or equal to) can be used in logical expressions. The SPSS manual should be consulted for a complete list of relational operators.

BCAGEMON *only* for cases where the Child is under 12 months of age. Such a listing is presented in Figure 1–3, for the first 10 cases meeting the age criterion. Note that the largest value for BCAGEMON now is 11—i.e., 11 months old. Cases where the Child is 1 year or older (e.g., case #1001 from Figure 1–2) are omitted in this listing. Statistical programs offer commands that can be used to select the appropriate cases.

Exercise. Using the data files for the NLSY data set, list the following variables for the first 10 cases where *the Child is **not** an only child,* using BCNSIBS to select cases:

ADID	ADINTMO	ADINTYR	BCRACE	BCGENDER	BCBIRTMO	BCBIRTYR	BCAGEMON
1012	3	86	3	1	10	85	4
1014	2	86	3	1	6	85	8
1019	5	86	3	1	9	85	8
1021	3	86	3	2	4	85	11
1022	4	86	3	1	9	85	7
1024	2	86	1	1	10	85	3
1041	5	86	3	2	6	85	10
1076	4	86	3	1	4	85	11
1101	2	86	3	2	12	85	2
1104	3	86	2	2	8	85	7

FIGURE 1–3. SPSS/PC PRINTOUT (LIST) FOR SELECTED VARIABLES FOR INFANTS UNDER 1 YEAR OLD

ADID, BCGENDER, BCAGE, BCNSIBS, BCSPACNG. When you have produced the listing for the five specified variables, check to make sure the selection process worked correctly by seeing if there are any only children (i.e., children for whom the value of BCNSIBS is 0) in the listing. Then use the printout and coding information in Appendix C to answer the following questions:

a. What is the ID number of the Child who has two siblings?
b. For the Child whose ID number is 1037, how many months separate the Child from his next younger sibling?
c. What is the ID number of the Child whose younger sibling is almost 4 years younger?
d. Of the 10 cases in the listing, how many of the Children have a sibling who is less than 2 years younger than they are?

B. INDEPENDENT COMPUTER EXERCISES

Use the NLSY data set to perform independent exercises based on the information discussed in Chapter 1 of the textbook. Some specific suggestions follow.

1. Find 10 (or more) variables in the NLSY data set that are of substantive interest to you. Write down a list of the variables by their variable names, and indicate their level of measurement.

2. For the 10 variables selected for Exercise B.1, produce a computer display of the basic variable information from the file, according to the procedure described in Exercise A.4. Compare the display you obtained with the display of these variables in Appendix C.

3. Choose 5 of the 10 variables selected for Exercise B.1 and instruct the computer to list the values of the first 15 cases, according to the procedure described in Exercise A.5. Be sure to include ADID when listing the variables.

4. List 15 cases for the remaining 5 variables (i.e., those not used in Exercise B.3) **but** list only cases where the mother was under age 20 when she first gave birth (selection variable = BMAGE1ST).

C. EXERCISES IN READING COMPUTER PRINTOUTS

The exercises in this section are based on printouts from a longitudinal study of over 2000 teenage mothers. Use the printouts to answer the questions included in the exercises.

1. Figure 1–4 presents a display of variables from the longitudinal study of teenage mothers. Using the printout, answer the following questions:

a. Which variables of those in Figure 1–4 have a missing values code of 99? Why do you think these variables used 99 rather than 9 for a missing values code?
b. Which variable of the six in the display is an ordinal-level variable?

c. In this data set, what code would be used to designate Puerto Rican women on the variable ETHNIC?

d. If a woman had not used birth control at her last sexual intercourse, what code would be assigned to LSTSEXBC?

e. Which variable that has a width of 2 *could* have had a width of 1 and still accommodated all coded values?

2. Figure 1–5 presents a listing of 7 variables for 15 cases, from the same longitudinal data set. Based on the printouts in Figures 1–4 and 1–5, answer the following questions:

a. What are the ID numbers of the white, non-Hispanic women in the listing?

b. How many women of the 15 listed are at high risk of clinical depression?

c. What are the ID numbers of women in the listing who had pregnancies that did not terminate (or have not yet terminated) in a live birth?

d. How many of the 15 women listed did not have a sexual partner at the time they were interviewed?

e. How many of the 15 women listed failed to use birth control the last time they had sexual intercourse?

```
Variable: ETHNIC          Label: ETHNIC GROUP
  Value labels follow   Type: Number  Width:  1  Dec: 0      Missing:      9.00
        1.00    WHITE, NON-HISP                 2.00   BLACK, NON-HISP
        3.00    MEXICAN                         4.00   PUERTO RICAN
        5.00    OTHER HISP                      6.00   AMER INDIAN/ALASKAN
        7.00    ASIAN

Variable: DEPRESS         Label: AT RISK OF CLINICL DEPRESSN-FRM CESD SCA
  Value labels follow   Type: Number  Width:  2  Dec: 0      Missing:      9.00
         .00    NOT AT RISK                     1.00   AT RISK
        2.00    AT HIGH RISK

Variable: PREGCNT         Label: NO OF PREGS AT BASELINE
  No value labels        Type: Number  Width:  2  Dec: 0     Missing:     99.00

Variable: BCNTRLN         Label: USING BIRTH CONTROL NOW
  Value labels follow   Type: Number  Width:  1  Dec: 0      Missing:      9.00
        1.00    YES, USING B.C.                 2.00   NO, NOT USING B.C.
        3.00    NO PARTNER                      4.00   NOT HAVING SEX

Variable: LSTSEXBC        Label: BIRTH CONTROL AT LAST SEX
  Value labels follow   Type: Number  Width:  1  Dec: 0      Missing:      9.00
        1.00    YES                             2.00   NO

Variable: LIVEBRTH        Label: NO. OF LIVE BIRTHS AT BASELINE
  No value labels        Type: Number  Width:  2  Dec: 0     Missing:     99.00
```

FIGURE 1–4. SPSS/PC PRINTOUT FOR EXERCISE C.1

ID1	ETHNIC	DEPRESS	PREGCNT	BCNTRLN	LSTSEXBC	LIVEBRTH
1	2	1	4	2	2	4
2	1	0	2	4	2	1
3	1	1	1	4	2	1
4	4	1	2	3	2	2
5	4	0	3	3	1	3
6	5	0	4	4	2	2
7	1	0	1	1	1	1
8	4	0	2	1	2	2
10	4	1	1	3	1	1
11	2	2	1	2	2	1
12	5	2	2	1	1	1
13	2	0	4	1	2	2
14	4	0	1	2	2	1
15	4	0	1	2	2	1
16	4	0	3	3	1	3

Number of cases read =   15   Number of cases listed =   15

FIGURE 1–5. SPSS/PC PRINTOUT FOR EXERCISE C.2

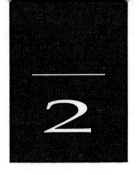

2

Univariate Statistics:
Tabulating and Displaying Data

A. DIRECTED COMPUTER EXERCISES

Appendixes A, B, and C of this Manual list all of the variables in the NLSY data set contained on the enclosed diskette. Perform the analyses described in the following exercises using the NLSY data set, and then answer the accompanying questions.

1. Using the data files for the NLSY data set, print a frequency distribution for the variable ADINTMO—the month in which the 1986 interview occurred.

When you have produced the frequency distribution for ADINTMO, use the printout to answer the following questions:

a. What is the *absolute* frequency of interviews completed in May? What is the *relative* frequency for that month? What is the *cumulative* relative frequency for May?
b. During which month did the highest percentage of 1986 interviews take place? What is the percentage?
c. During which month did the lowest percentage of 1986 interviews take place (excluding months in which *no* interviews were done)? What is the percentage?
d. By which month were 84.6% of the interviews completed?
e. For how many cases is there a missing value for the variable ADINTMO?

2. The variable BMHRSWK indicates the number of hours that the focal Child's mother worked in the week prior to the 1986 interview. Use the computer to generate a *grouped* frequency distribution for this variable, using a class interval of 10 (i.e., ≤ 10, 11-20, etc.).

SPSS Tip ───────────────────────────────

The basic SPSS/PC command that can be used to create frequency distributions is:

FREQUENCIES VARIABLES=VAR1, VAR2.

VAR1 and VAR2 are the names of the variables for which frequency distributions are desired. The TO convention can be used following the VARIABLES keyword to designate adjacent variables (e.g., VARIABLES=VAR1 TO VAR5). Various options for displaying the distributions (e.g., graphic displays) and for generating additional statistics are available in the FREQUENCIES program. The SPSS manual should be consulted.

When you have produced the grouped frequency distribution, use the printout to answer the following questions:

a. For the variable BMHRSWK, how many cases have valid (nonmissing) data? How many cases have missing data?
b. Using a class interval of 10, how many groups were created for BMHRSWK?
c. For the cases with valid data, what is the *absolute* frequency of women who worked 10 or fewer hours?
d. For the cases with valid data, what is the *relative* frequency of women who worked 31 to 40 hours?
e. What percentage of women worked *more than* 50 hours?

3. As indicated in the textbook, researchers examine frequency distributions when they are cleaning their data. Use the computer to generate a frequency distribution for the variable BMAGEYNG—the age of the mother's youngest child. Given the characteristics of the sample (see Part I, Section C.3), does the frequency distribution for BMAGEYNG suggest that there might be a wild code for this variable?

4. Using the computer, create a bar graph for the variable BCRACE (the Child's race/ethnicity). How many cases are in the racial/ethnic group that has the largest number of cases?

5. Using the computer, create a histogram for the variable BMAGE1ST (the mother's age when she first gave birth), displayed with percentages rather than absolute frequencies. Based on the histogram, answer the following questions:

SPSS Tip

The RECODE command can be used to group values into the desired class intervals prior to running the FREQUENCIES program. For example, to recode the Child's age in months to age in years, the following command would be used:

RECODE BCAGEMON (0 THRU 11=0)(12 THRU 23=1)
  (24 THRU 35=2)(36 THRU 47=3)(48 THRU 59=4)
  (60 THRU 71=5).

Note that the keyword THRU can be used to designate a range of adjacent values. In this case, for example, a Child whose original value for the variable BCAGEMON ranged from 0 to 11 would have it *all* recoded to zero, i.e., less than 1 year old.

---

a. Approximately what percentage of women gave birth when they were 25 years old?
b. At which ages did fewer than 5% of the mothers in the sample first give birth?
c. Describe the distribution of the BMAGE1ST variable in terms of modality and symmetry/skewness.

   6. Generate histograms for the following three variables: BCHHSIZE, BMAGEINT, and BMASP79. Based on the three histograms, answer the following questions:

a. Which of the three variables has a distinctly positive skew?
b. Which of the three variables is multimodal?
c. Which of the three variables most closely resembles a normal distribution?
d. Which variable could best be described as leptokurtic?

   7. *Background.* Variables in a data set are often manipulated to create new variables, as discussed in Section F of Part I. Researchers sometimes create variables to examine the cumulative extent of missing data across several variables prior to undertaking substantive analyses. Suppose, for example, that we had five key variables (VAR1, VAR2, VAR3, VAR4, and VAR5), some of which had missing values. We could create a new variable (sometimes called a **flag**) to count the number of missing values

SPSS Tip ———————————————————

The COUNT command can be used to create new variables in SPSS/PC. In the example of creating a missing values flag, the command would be:

COUNT MISSFLAG=VAR1 TO VAR5 (9).

Here the new variable is named MISSFLAG, and the variable would be set equal to the number of times the value of 9—the missing values code in this example—appeared for the five variables of interest, for each case in the file. The TO convention can be used on the COUNT command for variables that are adjacent in the file.

---

across all five variables. For example, if the first case in the data set had valid codes for VAR1 to VAR4 but had a missing values code for VAR5, the value of the new variable would be 1, because for that case there is one missing value. Across all cases in the file, the value of the new variable could range from 0 (for cases with no missing values) to 5 (for cases with all missing values for VAR1 to VAR5). We could then determine the size of the rectangular matrix for the five variables of interest—i.e., how many cases in the data set had **no** missing data for the five variables—by generating a frequency distribution for the new variable.

Exercise. In the NLSY data set, there are nine variables that indicate the mother's health-related behavior during her pregnancy with the focal Child (e.g., whether she took vitamins, smoked, etc.). Create a flag to count the number of missing values codes for the variables PRALCUSE to PRREDALC. Then generate a frequency distribution for the flag variable. For how many cases in the NLSY data set is there complete (non-missing) data? In other words, how many cases would be in a rectangular matrix for the variables of interest?

B. INDEPENDENT COMPUTER EXERCISES

Use the NLSY data set to perform independent analyses of the type described in Chapter 2 of the textbook. Some specific suggestions follow.

1. Identify five nominal-level or ordinal-level variables in the NLSY data set that are of substantive interest to you. Generate frequency distributions of these variables. Compare the 5 variables in terms of the number of valid cases and missing cases.

2. Identify five interval-level or ratio-level variables in the NLSY data set that are of substantive interest to you. Generate frequency distributions of these variables. Do any of the selected variables have any outliers?

3. Generate *grouped* frequency distributions of the same five variables used for Exercise B.2, using the ungrouped distribution to determine an appropriate class interval size. Check the printout to determine if the number of groups in the distribution conforms to the recommendations in Chapter 2 of the textbook.

4. For the five variables selected for Exercise B.2, generate histograms. Compare the five distributions in terms of modality, symmetry, and kurtosis. Which of the five distributions comes closest to approximating a normal distribution?

5. Create a variable that will count the number of missing values for the 10 variables identified in Exercises B.1 and B.2 for each case in the data set (see Exercise A.7). Generate a frequency distribution for this missing values flag. What is the size of the rectangular matrix that could be created for the 10 variables?

C. EXERCISES IN READING COMPUTER PRINTOUTS

The exercises in this section are based on printouts from a longitudinal study of over 2000 teenage mothers. Use the printouts to answer the questions included in the exercises.

1. Figure 2–1 presents a frequency distribution for the variable BCUSE, a measure of the young mothers' use of birth control at the time of the first interview. Using the printout in Figure 2–1, answer the following questions:

a. What is the total size of the sample in the data set?
b. What is the *absolute* frequency of young mothers who were regularly using birth control?

BCUSE   CURRENTLY USING BIRTH CONTROL?

Value Label	Value	Frequency	Percent	Valid Percent	Cum Percent
SEXUALLY ABSTINENT	1.00	377	17.9	21.0	21.0
REGULAR BC USE	2.00	791	37.6	44.0	64.9
IRREGULAR OR NO BC	3.00	631	30.0	35.1	100.0
	9.00	307	14.6	Missing	
	Total	2106	100.0	100.0	

Valid cases   1799   Missing cases   307

FIGURE 2–1. SPSS/PC PRINTOUT FOR EXERCISE C.1

c. What is the *relative* frequency of young women who were not using birth control or using it irregularly, based on valid cases only?

d. What is the *cumulative* relative frequency of young women who were not at risk of another pregnancy (i.e., were either abstinent or using birth control), based on valid cases only?

e. What code was used for missing values for the variable BCUSE? How many cases were missing? How many cases were *not* missing?

2. Figure 2–2 presents a condensed frequency distribution for the variable ESTEEM—the young mothers' scores on a self-esteem scale.[1] (Note that in the condensed format, percentages and cumulative percentages are for valid cases only and are rounded to the nearest whole number.) Use the printout to answer the following questions:

a. What was the *lowest* score on the ESTEEM variable in this sample? How many cases (absolute frequency) had this score?

b. What is the score at or below which 33% of the cases fell?

ESTEEM   SCORE ON SELF-ESTEEM SCALE

Value	Freq	Pct	Cum Pct	Value	Freq	Pct	Cum Pct	Value	Freq	Pct	Cum Pct
12.00	1	0	0	27.00	25	1	6	39.00	120	6	54
16.00	2	0	0	28.00	26	1	7	40.00	130	6	60
17.00	1	0	0	29.00	48	2	9	41.00	130	6	66
18.00	2	0	0	30.00	73	4	13	42.00	103	5	71
19.00	2	0	0	31.00	67	3	16	43.00	114	5	76
20.00	3	0	1	32.00	59	3	19	44.00	99	5	81
21.00	7	0	1	33.00	82	4	23	45.00	89	4	85
22.00	7	0	1	34.00	96	5	28	46.00	96	5	90
23.00	8	0	2	35.00	109	5	33	47.00	51	2	93
24.00	16	1	2	36.00	105	5	38	48.00	50	2	95
25.00	17	1	3	37.00	94	5	42	49.00	45	2	97
26.00	32	2	5	38.00	115	6	48	50.00	61	3	100

MISSING DATA

Value	Freq	Value	Freq	Value	Freq
.	18	99.00	3		

Valid cases   2085   Missing cases   21

FIGURE 2–2. SPSS/PC PRINTOUT FOR EXERCISE C.2

---

[1]The SPSS/PC commands that created the printout in Figure 2–2 are:

```
FREQUENCIES VARIABLES=ESTEEM
/FORMAT=CONDENSE.
```

SPSS Tip

A system-missing value is assigned by SPSS when there is a blank for a variable that has been defined as numeric. System-missing values are also assigned when a new variable is created via a transformation of an existing variable if the existing variable has a missing value. For example, if ESTEEM had been created by combining 10 variables (each representing one item on a 10-item scale) and a respondent had failed to complete one item, that person would have a system-missing value for ESTEEM.

c. What is the score with the highest absolute frequency? What is the relative frequency of that score?
d. In this example, there are two missing values codes—a *system-missing* value, designated by a period, and 99. How many cases were missing in total?
e. If you wanted to generate a grouped frequency distribution for the ESTEEM variable, what would be the most appropriate size for the class interval?

3. Figure 2–3 presents a histogram for the variable RGRADLVL. This variable indicates the young mothers' grade equivalent on a reading test. Use the printout to answer the following questions:

```
RGRADLVL   READING GRADE LEVEL

   COUNT        VALUE

       5        1.00  |X
      32        2.00  |XXXX
     121        3.00  |XXXXXXXXXXXXXX
     106        4.00  |XXXXXXXXXXXXX
     166        5.00  |XXXXXXXXXXXXXXXXXXXX
     222        6.00  |XXXXXXXXXXXXXXXXXXXXXXXXXXX
     264        7.00  |XXXXXXXXXXXXXXXXXXXXXXXXXXXXXXXX
     335        8.00  |XXXXXXXXXXXXXXXXXXXXXXXXXXXXXXXXXXXXXXXXXX
     246        9.00  |XXXXXXXXXXXXXXXXXXXXXXXXXXXXXXX
     168       10.00  |XXXXXXXXXXXXXXXXXXXX
      80       11.00  |XXXXXXXXXX
     339       12.00  |XXXXXXXXXXXXXXXXXXXXXXXXXXXXXXXXXXXXXXXXXX
                      I.........I.........I.........I.........I.........I
                      0         4         8        12        16        20
                                          Percent
```

FIGURE 2–3. SPSS/PC PRINTOUT FOR EXERCISE C.3

a. What is the absolute frequency—and the approximate relative frequency—of women reading at the eleventh grade level?
b. What is the reading grade level with the highest absolute frequency? What is that frequency?
c. How would the modality of the distribution be described?

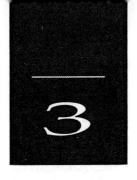

Univariate Statistics:
Central Tendency and Variability

A. DIRECTED COMPUTER EXERCISES

Appendixes A, B, and C of this manual list all of the variables in the NLSY data set contained on the enclosed diskette. Perform the analyses described in the following exercises using the NLSY data set, and then answer the accompanying questions.

1. Using the data files for the NLSY data set, generate a histogram for the variable BMAGEYNG (age of the mother's youngest child), displayed with percentages. Based on the histogram, answer the following questions:

a. What is the *mode* for the variable BMAGEYNG?
b. Describe the shape of the distribution in terms of symmetry/skewness.
c. Based on the distribution's shape, would you expect the mean to be greater than, less than, or equal to the mode?

2. Use the computer to compute the mean, median, and mode for the variables CDBODYP to CDPPVT, which are eight variables measuring aspects of the Child's development.

When you have produced the printout, use it to answer the following questions:

a. Rounding to one decimal place, what are the mean, median, and mode of the variable CDPPVT?
b. Based on the three indexes of central tendency, which two variables are especially likely to approximate a normal distribution? Why?

SPSS Tip

In SPSS/PC, subcommands of the FREQUENCIES program can be used to compute all three measures of central tendency. To print the central tendency statistics without the actual frequency distribution information, the following commands could be used:

```
FREQUENCIES VARIABLES=VAR1 TO VAR3
  /FORMAT=NOTABLE
  /STATISTICS=MEAN MEDIAN MODE.
```

The VARIABLES keyword identifies the variables of interest (here, VAR1, VAR2, and VAR3), the FORMAT subcommand instructs the computer to omit the frequency distribution table, and the STATISTICS subcommand identifies which descriptive statistics are desired.

---

c. For the variables CDBODYP, CDMEMSTO, and CDPIATRR, indicate whether the distribution is likely to be positively or negatively skewed.
d. Which of the eight variables has the largest number of missing cases? Which variable has the smallest number of missing cases?

3. Use the computer to compute the range, minimum value, maximum value, standard deviation, and variance for the variables CDBODYP to CDPPVT.
   Use the printout to answer the following questions:

a. Rounding to one decimal place, what are the range, standard deviation, and variance of the variable CDPPVT?
b. Which of the eight variables has the largest range? Does this variable also have the largest standard deviation?
c. Which variable has greater variability—CDPIATM or CDPIATRR?

4. Prepare a table of descriptive statistics suitable for presentation in a research report, based on printouts for the eight child development variables from Exercises A.2 and A.3. Include at least four different descriptive statistics, some of which are measures of central tendency and some of which are measures of variability.

5. Use the computer to generate measures of central tendency for the variable BMRELYNG (the religion in which the mother was raised). Answer the following questions based on the printout:

SPSS Tip ──────────────────────────────

In SPSS/PC, the FREQUENCIES program can also be used to compute measures of variability. The following commands could be used to produce the range, minimum and maximum, standard deviation, and variance, again without printing the full frequency distribution:

FREQUENCIES VARIABLES=VAR1 TO VAR3
 /FORMAT=NOTABLE
 /STATISTICS=RANGE MINIMUM MAXIMUM STDDEV VARIANCE.

The STATISTICS subcommand again identifies which descriptive statistics are desired. Note that if the STATISTICS subcommand specifies ALL, the computer will print the above indexes as well as the three indexes of central tendency and other descriptive statistics. (Other SPSS programs, such as DESCRIPTIVES, also can be used to generate some indexes of central tendency and variability.)

──

a. What is the mean value of BMRELYNG? Is this mean value meaningful? Why or why not?
b. Which of the indexes is meaningful? Why?

   6. Use the computer to compute standard scores with a mean of 0 and an SD of 1 for the variable CDMEMLOC; this will create a new variable, which can be called ZMEMLOC.
   For the first 10 cases in the file, *list* the values of CDMEMLOC and ZMEMLOC—and ADID—using the procedures described in exercise A.5 in Chapter 1 of this manual. Use the listing to answer the following questions:

a. What is the value of ZMEMLOC for case number 1001? Why does it have this value?
b. Verify that the standard score for case number 1005 was computed correctly. That is, using information on the mean and SD of CDMEMLOC from the printouts in Exercises A.2 and A.3, compute the standard score for this case.
c. In the listing, for which case is ZMEMLOC negative? Why is it negative?

   7. In 1980, about 96% of the mothers in the NLSY sample were administered an aptitude test known as the Armed Forces Qualification Test (the variable BMAFQT80). Use the computer to generate descriptive statistics for this variable. For the 4% of the sample

SPSS Tip

In SPSS/PC, subcommands of the DESCRIPTIVES program can be used to create standard scores with a mean of 0 and an *SD* of 1. These scores can then be used in subsequent analyses. For example, to create *Z* scores for a variable named FINLEXAM, we could use the following command:

DESCRIPTIVES VARIABLES=FINLEXAM (ZEXAM)
   /OPTIONS=3.

The VARIABLES keyword indicates which variable is of interest (here, FINLEXAM) and, in parentheses, what the name of the new standard score variable should be (ZEXAM).[1] The OPTIONS command specifies that standard scores should be computed; here the option number is 3, but the SPSS manual should be consulted to ascertain the appropriate number because the option numbers may be different in a different version of SPSS/PC.

---

with missing data on this variable, what value might be substituted in analyses involving this variable? Replace the missing values, and then recompute the descriptive statistics for BMAFQT80. To what extent did the statistics change after the substitution was made?

B. INDEPENDENT COMPUTER EXERCISES

Use the NLSY data set to perform independent analyses of the type described in Chapter 3 of the textbook. Some specific suggestions follow.

   1. Identify five interval-level or ratio-level variables in the NLSY data set that are of substantive interest to you. Use the computer to compute measures of central tendency and variability for these variables. Note any similarities and differences among the values of the three measures of central tendency.

   2. Prepare a table of descriptive statistics suitable for presentation in a research report, based on printouts for the five variables from Exercise B.1. Include at least four

---

[1]SPSS will assign a name to the standard score variable automatically if none is specified in parentheses: Z plus the first seven characters of the original variable name. Thus, the computer-assigned name here would have been ZFINLEXA.

SPSS Tip

In SPSS/PC, substitutions can be made using the IF or the RECODE commands. For example, suppose the missing value for the FINLEXAM variable was 99 and the value we wanted to use as a substitute was 45. *Either* of the following commands could be used:

IF (MISSING(FINLEXAM)) FINLEXAM=45.

RECODE FINLEXAM (99=45).

The IF command replaces old values of FINLEXAM with the value of 45 *if* the old value was specified as a missing value. The RECODE command changes any value of 99 (the missing code) to 45.

---

different descriptive statistics, some of which are measures of central tendency and some of which are measures of variability.

3. Use the computer to compute standard scores with a mean of 0 and an *SD* of 1 for at least one of the variables selected for Exercise B.1. Compute the three indexes of central tendency for the new standard score variable and compare the values of these indexes.

C. EXERCISES IN READING COMPUTER PRINTOUTS

The exercises in this section are based on printouts from a longitudinal study of over 2000 teenage mothers. Use the printouts to answer the questions included in these exercises.

1. Figure 3–1 presents a number of descriptive statistics for two variables from the longitudinal study. The variables represent the sample members' total number of pregnancies (PREGCNT) and number of live births (LIVEBRTH). Using the printout in Figure 3–1, answer the following questions:

a. For which of the two variables is there more missing data?
b. What is the mean number of pregnancies and live births?
c. The distributions of both variables are somewhat skewed. In which direction are they skewed? Which variable is more skewed?

```
PREGCNT   TOTAL NUMBER OF PREGNANCIES

Mean          1.893    Std err       .021    Median      2.000
Mode          1.000    Std dev       .957    Variance     .915
Kurtosis      -.425    S E Kurt      .107    Skewness     .784
S E Skew       .054    Range        3.000    Minimum     1.000
Maximum       4.000    Sum       3942.000

Valid cases    2082    Missing cases    24
```

- -

```
LIVEBRTH  NUMBER OF LIVE BIRTHS

Mean          1.434    Std err       .015    Median      1.000
Mode          1.000    Std dev       .676    Variance     .457
Kurtosis      2.190    S E Kurt      .107    Skewness    1.517
S E Skew       .054    Range        5.000    Minimum      .000
Maximum       5.000    Sum       2995.000

Valid cases    2088    Missing cases    18
```

FIGURE 3–1. SPSS/PC PRINTOUT FOR EXERCISE C.1

d. Had all the women in the sample had a pregnancy? Had they all given birth?
e. For which of the two variables was variability greater?

   2. Figure 3–2 presents a printout with several descriptive statistics for the two variables from Exercise C.1, plus two additional variables: AGE (the young mother's age) and AGE1BRTH (age when the mother first gave birth).[2] Use the printout to answer the following questions:

a. What was the *lowest* age at which a sample member had given birth?
b. What is the *range* of ages represented in the sample?
c. Compare the variability of AGE and AGE1BRTH.
d. Compare the means and SDs for PREGCNT and LIVEBRTH in Figures 3–1 and 3–2. What do you conclude?

   3. Figure 3–3 presents a printout with descriptive statistics for CESD (raw depression scale scores) and ZCESD (standard scores for the depression scale). Use the printout to answer the following questions:

---

[2]The SPSS/PC commands that created the printout in Figure 3–2 are:
      DESCRIPTIVES VARIABLES=PREGCNT,LIVEBIRTH,AGE,AGE1BRTH
      /STATISTICS=13.

```
Number of Valid Observations (Listwise) =      2082.00

Variable    Mean    Std Dev   Minimum   Maximum    N   Label

PREGCNT     1.89      .96        1         4      2082  TOTAL NUMBER OF PREG
LIVEBRTH    1.43      .68        0         5      2088  NUMBER OF LIVE BIRTH
AGE        18.85     1.38      16.00     22.00    2088  AGE AT THE TIME OF I
AGE1BRTH   17.33     1.39      10.03     21.87    2088  AGE WHEN 1ST GAVE BI
```

FIGURE 3–2. SPSS/PC PRINTOUT FOR EXERCISE C.2

a. Does the printout suggest that the standard scores were properly computed?
b. If a young mother in the sample had a raw score of 16 on the variable CESD, what would her score on ZCESD be, approximately?
c. If a young mother had a raw score of 0 on CESD, what would her score on ZCESD be?
d. What would the variance of ZCESD be?

```
Number of Valid Observations (Listwise) =      2106.00

Variable    Mean    Std Dev   Minimum   Maximum    N   Label

CESD       15.99    10.49       .00      57.00    2106  DEPRESSION SCALE RAW
ZCESD        .00     1.00    -1.52438   3.90864   2106  ZSCORE:   DEPRESSION
```

FIGURE 3–3. SPSS/PC PRINTOUT FOR EXERCISE C.3

Bivariate Description

A. DIRECTED COMPUTER EXERCISES

Appendixes A, B, and C of this Manual list all the variables in the NLSY data set contained on the enclosed diskette. Perform the analyses described in the following exercises using the NLSY data set, and then answer the accompanying questions.

1. Using the data files for the NLSY data set, crosstabulate the variables BCRACE and BCGENDER, displaying absolute and relative frequencies for each cell.

When you have produced the printout, use the contingency table to answer the following questions:

a. How many of the girls in the sample are Hispanic? How many boys are African-American?
b. What percentage of all the focal Children are non-Hispanic, non-African-American? What percentage of the Children are girls?
c. What percentage of girls are African-American? What percentage of boys are non-Hispanic, non-African-American?
d. What percentage of the Hispanic Children are boys? What percentage of the African-American Children are girls?
e. What percentage of the sample are Hispanic boys? What percentage of the sample are African-American girls? Which gender/racial group has the smallest percentage of cases?

2. Use the computer to generate the means for the variable PRBWT (the Child's weight at birth), broken down separately for male and female Children (BCGENDER).

SPSS Tip ——————————————————————

In SPSS/PC, two variables can be crosstabulated using the CROSSTABS command, as in the following example:

CROSSTABS TABLES=VAR1 BY VAR2
   /CELLS=COUNT ROW COLUMN TOTAL.

The CROSSTABS program crosstabulates the variables specified after TABLES=. The first variable, before the keyword BY, is the row variable in the contingency table, and the variable named after BY is the column variable. The CELLS= subcommand instructs the computer to present absolute frequencies (COUNT) and the row, column, and total percentages for each cell.

———————————————————————————————————————

When you have produced the printout, use it to answer the following questions:
a. What was the average birth weight for the entire sample?
b. On average, did boys or girls weigh more at birth? What was the average difference in birth weights, to one decimal place?
c. For which gender was birth weight variability greater?

SPSS Tip ——————————————————————

In SPSS/PC, means for an interval or ratio-level variable can be generated for all categories of a nominal-level variable using the MEANS command, as in the following example:

MEANS TABLES=VAR1 BY VAR2.

The MEANS program computes means and standard deviations for the variable named before the keyword BY, for every level of the variable named after BY.

———————————————————————————————————————

d. For how many cases was birth weight information missing? What percentage of the sample did this constitute?

3. Produce a scatterplot graphing the relationship between a focal Child's height (HLHEIGHT) and weight (HLWEIGHT).

When you have produced the printout, use the plot to answer the following questions:

a. Describe the nature of the relationship between the two variables, based on the scatterplot.
b. How many times were there values of the Child's height and weight that were the same for more than 35 cases?
c. The most extreme outlier on the BCHEIGHT variable was a Child who was (about) how tall?
d. The most extreme outlier on the BCWEIGHT variable was a Child who weighed (about) how much?

4. Use the computer to generate a correlation matrix with the following variables: BCAGEMON (Child's age in months), BCAGE (Child's age in years), HLHEIGHT (Child's height), and HLWEIGHT (Child's weight). Use listwise deletion; i.e., include in the matrix only cases with valid (nonmissing) data for all variables in the matrix.

When you have produced the printout, use the matrix to answer the following questions:

SPSS Tip

In SPSS/PC, the command for producing a scatterplot is PLOT, as in the following example:

PLOT PLOT=VAR1 WITH VAR2.

This command will create a scatterplot in which the first-named variable (here, VAR1) is graphed on the vertical axis, and the variable following the keyword WITH is graphed on the horizontal axis. The printout shows the frequency of values at the intersection of two plotted variables. By default, the actual frequency is shown for frequencies up to 9, while for frequencies between 10 and 35, an alphabetic symbol is used (A = 10, B = 11, etc.). For frequencies 36 and greater, an asterisk is used.

SPSS Tip ————————————

In SPSS/PC, Pearson's product-moment correlation coefficients can be generated using the CORRELATIONS program, as in the following example:

CORRELATIONS VARIABLES=VAR1, VAR2, VAR3.

This command will compute a correlation matrix for all variables specified. By default, cases that have missing values for any named variable will be excluded. (For pairwise deletion, which excludes cases with missing values on a pair-by-pair basis, a separate option must be specified.)

———————————————————————————

a. What is the value of the correlation coefficient between BCAGE and BCAGEMON?
b. For which two variables is the correlation coefficient .8932?
c. Is there a stronger correlation between a Child's age and his/her weight or between his/her age and height?
d. On how many cases was the correlation matrix based?

B. INDEPENDENT COMPUTER EXERCISES

Use the NLSY data set to perform independent analyses of the type described in Chapter 4 of the textbook. Some specific suggestions follow.

1. Identify five nominal-level variables in the NLSY data set that are of substantive interest to you. Crosstabulate them all by the Child's gender (or by another nominal-level variable of interest to you).

2. Identify five interval-level or ratio-level variables in the NLSY data set that are of substantive interest to you. Use the computer to generate means for all five variables, broken down by the Child's gender (or another nominal-level variable of interest to you).

3. Identify two interval- or ratio-level variables that you suspect are correlated with each other. Use the computer to produce a scatterplot of the two variables. Then plot two variables that you suspect are *not* correlated with each other. Based on the plots, are your suspicions about the relationships confirmed?

4. Using the variables identified in Exercise B.3, create a correlation matrix. Compare what you learned about the relationship among variables from the scatterplots and the correlation matrix.

C. EXERCISES IN READING COMPUTER PRINTOUTS

The exercises in this section are based on printouts from a longitudinal study of over 2000 teenage mothers. Use the printouts to answer the questions included in the exercises.

1. Figure 4–1 presents a printout of a contingency table for two variables from the longitudinal study. The variables indicate the mothers' total number of miscarriages (MISCARR), by whether or not they had obtained a high school diploma (DIPLOMA). Using the printout in Figure 3–1, answer the following questions:

a. How many young mothers had no miscarriages? What percentage of the sample with valid data was this?
b. How many young mothers had obtained a high school diploma? What percentage of the sample with valid data was this?
c. Among the mothers with one miscarriage, what percentage had a high school diploma? What percentage of the total sample had one miscarriage *and* had obtained a diploma?
d. Among the mothers with a diploma, what percentage had 3 miscarriages? What percentage of the total sample had a diploma *and* had three miscarriages?
e. How many cases had missing data? Can you tell from the printout whether the data were missing for DIPLOMA or MISCARR (or both)?

2. Figure 4–2 presents a printout with the means and standard deviations for ESTEEM (scores on a self-esteem scale), broken down by whether or not the young mother has a high school diploma. Use the printout to answer the following questions:

```
DIPLOMA  HAS A HIGH SCHOOL DIPLOMA?  by  MISCARR  NUMBER OF MISCARRIAGES

                    MISCARR                        Page 1 of 1
            Count
            Row Pct
            Col Pct                                     Row
            Tot Pct     .00|   1.00|   2.00|   3.00| Total
  DIPLOMA   --------+--------+--------+--------+--------+
              .00       735     260      39      12     1046
   NO                  70.3    24.9     3.7     1.1     63.2
                       62.7    65.2    60.9    63.2
                       44.4    15.7     2.4      .7
                    +--------+--------+--------+--------+
             1.00       437     139      25       7      608
   YES                 71.9    22.9     4.1     1.2     36.8
                       37.3    34.8    39.1    36.8
                       26.4     8.4     1.5      .4
                    +--------+--------+--------+--------+
            Column     1172     399      64      19     1654
            Total      70.9    24.1     3.9     1.1    100.0

Number of Missing Observations:   452
```

FIGURE 4–1. SPSS/PC PRINTOUT FOR EXERCISE C.1

```
Summaries of    ESTEEM      SCORE ON SELF-ESTEEM SCALE
By levels of    DIPLOMA     HAS A HIGH SCHOOL DIPLOMA?

Variable      Value Label                    Mean      Std Dev     Cases

For Entire Population                       38.3458    6.5340      2085

DIPLOMA          .00  NO                    38.1097    6.5636      1276
DIPLOMA         1.00  YES                   38.7182    6.4735       809

   Total Cases =     2106
Missing Cases =        21 OR   1.0 PCT.
--------------------------------------------------------------------
```

FIGURE 4–2. SPSS/PC PRINTOUT FOR EXERCISE C.2

a. What was the mean score on the self-esteem scale for the total sample of young mothers? What was the *SD*?
b. How many cases was the overall mean based on? How many cases overall were missing?
c. Who had the higher self-esteem scores, on average—women with or women without a high school diploma?

3. Figure 4–3 presents a printout with a correlation matrix for five variables: CESD (depression scale scores), ESTEEM (self-esteem scale scores), INTERNAL (internal-external Locus of Control Scale scores), SUPSATIS (scores on a satisfaction with social support scale), and DLC (scores on the Difficult Life Circumstances Scale). Use the printout to answer the following questions:

a. With which variable is CESD most strongly correlated? With which variable is CESD most weakly correlated?
b. Which is the stronger relationship—the correlation between DLC and ESTEEM or the correlation between SUPSATIS and INTERNAL?
c. Which two variables are negatively correlated with SUPSATIS?
d. What is the weakest correlation in the matrix?

```
Correlations:  CESD       ESTEEM     INTERNAL   SUPSATIS    DLC

   CESD      1.0000     -.2965**   -.1796**   -.1468**    .4338**
   ESTEEM    -.2965**   1.0000      .3985**    .2051**   -.1170**
   INTERNAL  -.1796**    .3985**   1.0000      .0940**   -.0435
   SUPSATIS  -.1468**    .2051**    .0940**   1.0000     -.0649*
   DLC        .4338**   -.1170**   -.0435     -.0649*    1.0000

N of cases:  2044        2-tailed Signif:  * - .01  ** - .001
```

FIGURE 4–3. SPSS/PC PRINTOUT FOR EXERCISE C.3

Statistical Inference

A. DIRECTED COMPUTER EXERCISES

Appendixes A, B, and C of this Manual list all the variables in the NLSY data set contained on the enclosed diskette. Perform the analyses described in the following exercises using the NLSY data set, and then answer the accompanying questions.

1. The following are null hypotheses concerning some of the variables in the NLSY data set. State two alternative hypotheses (nondirectional and directional) for each:

a. The mean population birth weight is 7.0 pounds (112 ounces.):

H_0: $\mu_{PRBWT} = 112.0$

b. The mean population age at first birth is 22 years:

H_0: $\mu_{BMAGE1ST} = 22.0$

c. The mean population household size is four people:

H_0: $\mu_{BCHHSIZE} = 4.0$

2. Use the computer to generate information about the mean and the standard error of the mean for the variables MDALCAGE (age at which the mother began to drink alcohol regularly) and MDCIGAGE (age at which the mother first tried a cigarette). Using the tabled value of t = 1.96 for = .05, construct a 95% confidence interval around both means.

SPSS Tip

In SPSS/PC, the FREQUENCIES program, described in Chapters 2 and 3, can be used to generate the mean and *SEM* (/STATISTICS=MEAN SEMEAN). Alternatively, the DESCRIPTIVES program can be used, as in the following example:

```
DESCRIPTIVES VARIABLES=VAR1 TO VAR3
    /STATISTICS=1,2.
```

This program generates descriptive statistics for the specified variables; the statistics correspond to numerical codes. In the version of SPSS/PC we used, 1 was the code for the mean and 2 was the code for the *SEM*. Consult the SPSS/PC manual to verify the appropriate codes for the version you are using.

---

3. Using the tabled value of $t = 2.58$ for $= .01$, construct a 99% confidence interval around the two means in exercise A.2. Use the two sets of confidence intervals to answer the following questions:

a. Does the age of 14 fall within or outside the 99% confidence interval for the mother's mean age of regular alcohol use?
b. Does the age of 14 fall within or outside the 99% confidence interval for the mother's mean age of first trying a cigarette?
c. What is the *range* of the 95% confidence interval for MDCIGAGE? How much larger is the range for the 99% confidence interval?
d. For which of the two variables is the 99% confidence larger? Why?

4. Use the computer to test the three null hypotheses in Exercise A.1, using a one-sample *t*-test.

When you have generated the *t*-tests, use the printout to answer the following questions:

a. At the .05 significance level, which of the null hypotheses are accepted and which are rejected?
b. What is the value of *t* for the *t*-test of the first hypothesis (for PRBWT)?
c. What is the standard deviation for the created variable for the hypothesized population value of BMAGE1ST (i.e., HYP@AGE1)?
d. How many degrees of freedom are there for the third *t*-test (for BCHHSIZE)?

SPSS Tip

In SPSS/PC, one-sample *t*-tests can be performed using the T-TEST program. However, before running the program, a new variable must be created for each test. The new variable designates the value of hypothesized population mean. For example, suppose we were testing the null hypothesis that the mean height of a sample of women was 65 inches. We would need to create a variable with a mean of 65 against which *actual* heights would be compared:

COMPUTE HYP@HITE=65.

This command sets the value of a new variable (HYP@HITE) equal to 65 for all cases in the sample, and thus the mean of this variable *must* be 65. Now we can instruct the computer to do the *t*-test:

T-TEST PAIRS=HEIGHT HYP@HITE.

This command instructs the computer to compute a *t*-test in which actual heights (HEIGHT) are compared to a hypothesized population height (HYP@HITE) of 65.

---

5. If people were born at random times throughout the year (i.e., equally likely to be born in January, February, etc.), you would expect that the mean for a birth month variable would be 6.5 (months 1 to 12 divided in half is 6.5). Use a one-sample *t*-test with the variable BCBIRTMO (month of the Child's birth) to test whether birth months are randomly distributed. Answer the following questions based on the printout:

a. What is the mean birth month of the Children? What is the *SD*?
b. What is the value of *t* for the *t*-test comparing the actual birth month to the hypothesized value of 6.5?
c. Is this *t* statistically significant? At what level?
d. What can you conclude based on this test?

B. INDEPENDENT COMPUTER EXERCISES

Use the NLSY data set to perform independent analyses of the type described in Chapter 5 of the textbook. Some specific suggestions follow.

1. Identify five interval-level or ratio-level variables in the NLSY data set that are of substantive interest to you. Make predictions about what the mean value of those variables might be. State the null and alternative hypotheses corresponding to your predictions.

2. Use the computer to generate information about the mean and the standard error of the mean for five interval-level or ratio-level variables in the NLSY data set that are of substantive interest to you. Using the tabled value of $t = 1.96$ for = .05, construct a 95% confidence interval around all means.

3. Use the computer to perform a one-sample t-test to test the five null hypotheses generated for Exercise B.1. Which of the five null hypotheses are accepted and which are rejected at the .05 level of significance? At the .01 level of significance?

C. EXERCISES IN READING COMPUTER PRINTOUTS

The exercises in this section are based on printouts from a longitudinal study of over 2000 teenage mothers. Use the printouts to answer the questions included in the exercises.

1. Figure 5–1 presents a printout of a t-test that tested the null hypothesis that the mean number of abortions the young mothers had was zero, i.e.:

H_0: $\mu_{ABORTS} = 0.0$

H_1: $\mu_{ABORTS} \neq 0.0$

The hypothesized population mean is designated by the variable named HYP@ABOR. Use the printout in Figure 5–1 to answer the following questions:

—t-tests for paired samples—

Variable	Number of pairs	Corr	2-tail Sig	Mean	SD	SE of Mean
ABORTS NUMBER OF ABORTIONS				.4490	.826	.018
	2098	.	.			
HYP@ABOR				.0000	.000	.000

Mean	Paired Differences SD	SE of Mean	t-value	df	2-tail Sig
.4490	.826	.018	24.91	2097	.000
95% CI (.414, .484)					

FIGURE 5–1. SPSS/PC PRINTOUT FOR EXERCISE C.1

a. What was the mean number of actual abortions for the young mothers? What is the standard deviation?

b. What is the *SEM* for the variable ABORTS? Using the tabled value of $t = 1.96$ for $\alpha = .05$, construct a 95% confidence interval around the mean for ABORTS.

c. What is the value of t for the t-test comparing the actual number of abortions (ABORTS) to the hypothesized value of 0.0 (HYP@ABOR)?

d. Is this t statistically significant? At what level?

2. Figure 5–2 presents a printout with information on the mean and *SEM* for four variables:

- EARNTOT (total earnings of the young mother in the prior month, among those with any earnings from employment)
- WELF$MO (amount of welfare mother received in the prior month, for those receiving welfare)
- FS$MO (dollar value of food stamps mother received in the prior month, for those receiving food stamps)
- HWAGEA (hourly wage received by mother in the most recently held job, for those with any work experience)

The first panel of the printout presents the means and *SEMs* for white women, while the second panel presents comparable information for nonwhite women in the sample. Use the printout in Figure 5–2 to address the following questions:

```
DESCRIPTIVES FOR WHITES ONLY

Number of Valid Observations (Listwise) =        80.00

Variable      Mean S.E. Mean      N  Label

EARNTOT      582.29      36.66    140  TOTAL ANNUAL EARNINGS PREVIOUS MONTH
WELF$MO      384.70       7.08    444  AMOUNT OF WELFARE CHECK PRIOR MONTH
FS$MO        191.29       3.61    369  AMOUNT OF FOOD STAMPS PRIOR MONTH
HWAGEA         4.90        .16    266  HOURLY WAGE, MOST RECENT JOB
-----------------------------------------------------------------------

DESCRIPTIVES FOR NONWHITES ONLY

Number of Valid Observations (Listwise) =       220.00

Variable      Mean S.E. Mean      N  Label

EARNTOT      627.76      26.58    309  TOTAL ANNUAL EARNINGS PREVIOUS MONTH
WELF$MO      397.93       4.08   1575  AMOUNT OF WELFARE CHECK PRIOR MONTH
FS$MO        189.84       1.88   1423  AMOUNT OF FOOD STAMPS PRIOR MONTH
HWAGEA         4.99        .09    715  HOURLY WAGE, MOST RECENT JOB
-----------------------------------------------------------------------
```

FIGURE 5–2. SPSS/PC PRINTOUT FOR EXERCISE C.2

a. How many white women in the sample had any earnings in the prior month? How many nonwhite women had earnings?
b. Construct a 95% confidence interval around the means for WELF$MO for the two groups of women, using the value of 1.96 for *t*. Is there any overlap in the two confidence intervals? Does the dollar amount of $395.00 fall within or outside the 95% confidence interval for the mother's average monthly welfare amount for either or both groups?
c. On average, did whites or nonwhites receive a higher amount for food stamps in the prior month? What was the average difference?
d. For which group is the *SEM* for HWAGEA larger? Why might that be?

Testing the Difference Between Two Means: The Two-Sample t-Test

A. DIRECTED COMPUTER EXERCISES

Appendixes A, B, and C of this Manual list all the variables in the NLSY data set contained on the enclosed diskette. Perform the analyses described in the following exercises using the NLSY data set, and then answer the accompanying questions.

    1. The following are null hypotheses involving a comparison between two independent groups in the NLSY data set. State two alternative hypotheses (nondirectional and directional) for each:

a. Women who get prenatal care in the first trimester have infants whose birth weights are the same as those whose mothers have no prenatal care in the first trimester.

    H_0: $\mu_{\text{PRBWT for PRTRIM1(yes)}} = \mu_{\text{PRBWT for PRTRIM1(no)}}$

b. Women who reduce their caloric intake during pregnancy gain the same amount of weight during the pregnancy as women who do not:

    H_0: $\mu_{\text{PRWTGAIN for PRCALORI(yes)}} = \mu_{\text{PRWTGAIN for PRCALORI(no)}}$

c. The number of weeks of gestation is the same for infants born by cesarean as for those not born by cesarean:

    H_0: $\mu_{\text{PRGESTAT for PRCESAR(yes)}} = \mu_{\text{PRGESTAT for PRCESAR(no)}}$

SPSS Tip ———————————————————

In SPSS/PC, two-sample *t*-tests for independent groups can be performed using the T-TEST program. The following commands can be used:

T-TEST GROUPS=GENDER (1,2)
  /VARIABLES=VAR1 TO VAR3.

This command instructs the computer to compute *t*-tests in which the independent variable (GROUPS=) is GENDER. Cases with GENDER coded 1 will be contrasted to cases with GENDER coded 2 with respect to three dependent variables: VAR1, VAR2, and VAR3.

———————————————————————————————

2. Use the computer to perform *t*-tests to test the three null hypotheses from Exercise A.1.

Use the printouts from the *t*-tests to answer the following questions:

a. What are the values of the *t* statistics for the three tests, for the pooled variance (equal variance) formula?
b. At the .05 level of significance for a two-tailed test, which of the three null hypotheses is rejected?
c. At the .01 level of significance for a two-tailed test, which of the three null hypotheses is rejected?
d. Are there any *t*-tests for which the null hypotheses must be accepted at the .05 level for a two-tailed test, but that can be rejected at the .05 level for a one-tailed test? If so, which one?
e. For which of the three *t*-tests (if any) is it necessary to use the separate variance formula?
f. Assuming a .05 level of significance, state your conclusion based on the *t*-test for each of the three hypotheses, as it might be written for a research report.

3. The following are null hypotheses involving a dependent groups situation for variables in the NLSY data set. State two alternative hypotheses (nondirectional and directional) for each:

a. The average number of times a woman is suspended from school while she was a student is the same as the average number of times she is expelled from school:

H_0: $\mu_{BMSUSP80} = \mu_{BMEXPL80}$

b. Among women who have ever smoked and who have ever used alcohol regularly, the average age the women first tried a cigarette is the same as the average age they began to drink regularly:

H_0: $\mu_{MDCIGAGE} = \mu_{MDALCAGE}$

c. Women's educational aspirations (number of years of education wanted) is equal to their educational attainment (number of years of education completed) 7 years later:

H_0: $\mu_{BMASP79} = \mu_{BMHIGRAD}$

4. Use the computer to perform *t*-tests to test the three null hypotheses from Exercise A.3.[1]

Use the printouts from the *t*-tests to answer the following questions:

a. What are the values of the *t* statistic for the three tests, for the pooled variance (equal variance) formula?
b. At the .05 level of significance for a two-tailed test, which of the three null hypotheses is rejected?

SPSS Tip

In SPSS/PC, two-sample *t*-tests for dependent groups can be performed using the T-TEST program. The following command can be used:

T-TEST PAIRS=VAR1 VAR2.

This command instructs the computer to compute a dependent groups *t*-test in which VAR1 is compared to VAR2 for all cases with valid data for both variables.

---

[1] Note that one of the codes for the variable BMHIGRAD is 95, for those whose educational level is ungraded. Cases with a value of 95 for BMHIGRAD should be excluded from the analysis. In SPSS/PC, this can be accomplished by using the SELECT IF or PROCESS IF command prior to the T-TEST command.

c. At the .01 level of significance for a two-tailed test, which of the three null hypotheses is rejected?

d. Are there any *t*-tests for which the null hypotheses must be accepted at the .05 level for a two-tailed test, but that can be rejected at the .05 level for a one-tailed test? If so, which one?

e. What is the mean difference for each of the three tests and what is the 95% confidence interval around each mean difference?

f. Assuming a .05 level of significance for a two-tailed test, state your conclusion based on the *t*-test for each of the three hypotheses, as it might be written for a research report.

B. INDEPENDENT COMPUTER EXERCISES

Use the NLSY data set to perform independent analyses of the type described in Chapter 6 of the textbook. Some specific suggestions follow.

1. Identify a dichotomous variable in the NLSY data set that is of substantive interest to you. (Note that new dichotomous variables can be created by manipulating the data in certain ways; for example, the variable PRBWT—infant's actual birth weight in ounces—can be used to create a dichotomous variable distinguishing low-birth-weight and normal-birth-weight infants.) Using the selected dichotomous variable as your independent variable, make predictions about the mean values for three dependent variables that are of substantive interest to you and that are meaningful in terms of the independent variable. State the null and alternative hypotheses corresponding to your predictions. Remember that the dependent variables for this exercise must be interval- or ratio-level variables.

2. Use the computer to perform two-sample *t*-tests for independent groups to test the three null hypotheses generated for Exercise B.1. Which of the three null hypotheses are accepted and which are rejected at the .05 level of significance? At the .01 level of significance? (Remember to use the unequal—separate—variance formula if appropriate.) Assuming a .05 level of significance for a two-tailed test, state your conclusions based on the t-tests for the three hypotheses, as they might be written for a research report, and prepare a table summarizing the results.

C. EXERCISES IN READING COMPUTER PRINTOUTS

The exercises in this section are based on printouts from a longitudinal study of over 2000 teenage mothers. Use the printouts to answer the questions included in the exercises.

1. Figure 6–1 presents an SPSS/PC printout for a *t*-test that tests the null hypothesis that women who had a new pregnancy between the baseline interview and a follow-up interview conducted 18 months later had the same average scores on a scale that measured mastery/self-efficacy as women who did not have a subsequent pregnancy:

```
t-tests for independent samples of  NEWPREG    PREGNANT AFTER BASELINE?
```

| | Number | | | |
Variable	of Cases	Mean	SD	SE of Mean
MASTERY SCORE ON MASTERY/SELF-EFFICACY SCALE				
NO	940	22.3096	3.401	.111
YES	1166	21.8937	3.406	.100

```
Mean Difference = .4159

Levene's Test for Equality of Variances: F= .031   P= .860
```

| | t-test for Equality of Means | | | | 95% |
Variances	t-value	df	2-Tail Sig	SE of Diff	CI for Diff
Equal	2.79	2104	.005	.149	(.123, .709)
Unequal	2.79	2011.43	.005	.149	(.123, .709)

FIGURE 6–1. SPSS/PC PRINTOUT FOR EXERCISE C.1

H_0: $\mu_{\text{MASTERY for NEWPREG(yes)}} = \mu_{\text{MASTERY for NEWPREG(no)}}$

H_1: $\mu_{\text{MASTERY for NEWPREG(yes)}} \neq \mu_{\text{MASTERY for NEWPREG(no)}}$

Use the printout in Figure 6–1 to answer the following questions:

a. How many young women in the sample had a subsequent pregnancy? How many did not?
b. What is the mean Mastery Scale score for women who had a subsequent pregnancy, and for those who did not? (Note: Higher scores indicate a higher perceived sense of mastery/self-efficacy).
c. What is the value of the *t* statistic for the pooled variance (equal variance) formula? What is the value of the *t* statistic for the separate (unequal) variance formula?
d. Should the pooled variance or separate variance estimate of *t* be used? Why?
e. At the .05 level of significance for a two-tailed test, can the null hypotheses be rejected? What is the exact probability level?
f. Assuming a .05 level of significance, state your conclusion based on the *t*-test, as it might be written for a research report.
g. Compute the value of r_{pb} for the relationship between Mastery Scale scores and the incidence of a pregnancy after baseline.

2. Figure 6–2 presents an SPSS/PC printout for a dependent groups *t*-test that tests the null hypothesis that the young mothers' average depression scale score at the time

—t-tests for paired samples—

Variable	Number of pairs	Corr	2-tail Sig	Mean	SD	SE of Mean
BASECESD DEPRESSION SCORE AT BASELINE				18.1088	10.253	.224
	2086	.420	.000			
CESD DEPRESSION SCORE 1ST FOLLOWUP				15.9971	10.503	.230

Paired Differences Mean	SD	SE of Mean	t-value	df	2-tail Sig
2.1117	11.179	.245	8.63	2085	.000
95% CI (1.632, 2.592)					

FIGURE 6–2. SPSS/PC PRINTOUT FOR EXERCISE C.2

of the baseline interview (BASECESD) is the same as their average depression scale score at the time of the follow-up interview 18 months later (CESD):

H_0: $\mu_{BASECESD} = \mu_{CESD}$

H_1: $\mu_{BASECESD} \neq \mu_{CESD}$

Use the printout in Figure 6–2 to answer the following questions:

a. For how many women was there a valid depression scale score at both points in time?
b. What is the mean Depression Scale score for the young women at baseline, and what was the mean score at the time of the 18-month follow-up interview? (Note: Higher scores reflect higher levels of depression.)
c. What is the mean difference score on the depression scale at the two points in time? What is the 95% confidence interval for the mean paired difference?
d. What is the value of the t statistic? What are the degrees of freedom for the test?
e. At the .05 level of significance for a two-tailed test, can the null hypotheses be rejected? What is the exact probability level?
f. Assuming a .05 level of significance, state your conclusion based on the t-test, as it might be written for a research report.

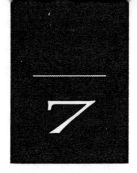

Analysis of Variance

A. DIRECTED COMPUTER EXERCISES

Appendixes A, B, and C of this Manual list all the variables in the NLSY data set contained on the enclosed diskette. Perform the analyses described in the following exercises using the NLSY data set, and then answer the accompanying questions.

1. The variable PRREDSMO in the NLSY data set is a 3-category variable that indicates the mother's smoking habits and reduction in smoking during her pregnancy with the focal Child: 0 is the code for women who were smokers and who did not reduce smoking during the pregnancy; 1 is the code for smokers who *did* reduce their smoking; and 4 is the code for nonsmokers. Perform an analysis of variance to test the null hypothesis that an infant's birthweight is unrelated to his or her mother's smoking habits during the pregnancy, i.e.:

$$H_0: \mu_{\text{PRBWT for PRREDSMO(0)}} = \mu_{\text{PRBWT for PRREDSMO(1)}} = \mu_{\text{PRBWT for PRREDSMO(4)}}$$

Use the printout from the analysis of variance to answer the following questions:

a. How many women in the sample were smokers who continued to smoke at prepregnancy levels? How many smokers reduced their smoking during the pregnancy? How many women were nonsmokers?
b. For which smoking group was the mean birth weight the highest? For which smoking group was birth weight the lowest?
c. For the ANOVA, what was the mean square between groups? The mean square within groups?

SPSS Tip ——————————————————————————

In SPSS/PC, a one-way analysis of variance can be performed via the MEANS, ONEWAY, and ANOVA programs. Here are the commands for the MEANS program:

MEANS TABLES=DV BY IV
  /STATISTICS=1.

This command instructs the computer to compute means for the dependent variable named DV separately for groups defined by the independent variable named IV. The STATISTICS=1 subcommand is the instruction to perform the analysis of variance.

——————————————————————————————————————

d. What was the value of the *F* statistic? What were the degrees of freedom?
e. Was the value of *F* statistically significant at the .05 level? What was the exact probability value?
f. What was the value of eta^2?
g. Assuming a .05 level of significance, state your conclusion based on the ANOVA, as it might be written for a research report.

2. Determine the *nature* of the relationship between PRBWT (infant's birth weight) and PRREDSMO (mother's smoking habits during pregnancy) from Exercise A.1 by using the computer to perform multiple comparison tests. Use Fisher's LSD test, the Sheffé test, and Tukey's test.

Use the printout from the multiple comparison tests to answer the following questions:

a. Are the results from the three multiple comparison tests the same, or do different tests lead to different conclusions?
b. According to the LSD test, which smoking groups (if any) are significantly different from each other with regard to infants' birth weight? At what level of significance?
c. According to the Tukey test, which smoking groups (if any) are *not* significantly different from each other with regard to infants' birth weight?
d. Assuming a .05 level of significance, state your conclusion based on the LSD multiple comparison test, as it might be written for a research report.

SPSS Tip

In SPSS/PC, multiple comparison tests are performed using the ONEWAY program, as in the following example:

```
ONEWAY DV BY IV (1,3)
  /RANGES=LSD
  /RANGES=TUKEY
  /RANGES=SHEFFE
  /OPTIONS=6
  /STATISTICS=1.
```

The ONEWAY command instructs the computer to perform a one-way ANOVA for the dependent variable DV. The independent variable IV has a minimum value of 1 and a maximum value of 3, shown in parentheses. The next three subcommands (/RANGES=) indicate that three multiple comparison tests should be performed (LSD, TUKEY, and SHEFFE); other multiple comparison tests are available. The OPTIONS=6 subcommand instructs the computer to use the value labels associated with the independent variable to label the groups being compared. Finally, the STATISTICS=1 subcommand instructs the computer to print group descriptive statistics (mean, SD, SEM, etc.).

---

3. The variable BCRACE in the NLSY data set is a four-category variable that indicates the child's race/ethnicity; 1 is the code for Hispanic children, 2 is the code for African-American children, and 3 is the code for non-Hispanic, non-African-American children. Perform a one-way analysis of variance to test the null hypothesis that—*among 4-year-old Children only*[1]—the Child's height (HLHEIGHT) is unrelated to his or her race/ethnicity; i.e.:

H_0: $\mu_{\text{HLHEIGHT for BCRACE(1)}}$ = $\mu_{\text{HLHEIGHT for BCRACE(2)}}$ = $\mu_{\text{HLHEIGHT for BCRACE(3)}}$

---

[1] Use the variable BCAGE to select cases. As a reminder for those using SPSS/PC, either the PROCESS IF or SELECT IF command can be used to restrict the analysis to 4-year-olds.

Also perform the LSD multiple comparison test *if* the ANOVA is statistically significant. Use the printout from the analysis of variance (and, if appropriate, the LSD test) to answer the following questions:

a. How many Children in the sample were 4-year-olds who had valid information on height in the data set?
b. Which group of 4-year-old Children was tallest, on average? Which group was shortest, on average?
c. For the ANOVA, what was the sum of squares between groups? The sum of squares within groups? The total sum of squares?
d. What was the value of the *F* statistic? What were the degrees of freedom?
e. Was the value of *F* statistically significant at the .05 level? What was the exact probability value?
f. If the ANOVA was significant, which groups were different from each other at statistically significant levels?
g. Assuming a .05 level of significance, state your conclusion based on the ANOVA and multiple comparison test, as it might be written for a research report.

   4. Using the same dependent variable as in Exercise A.3 (HLHEIGHT), perform a two-way ANOVA, with BCRACE (Child's race/ethnicity) as one independent variable and BCGENDER (Child's gender) as the other—*again, for 4-year-old Children only.*
   Use the printout from the analysis of variance to answer the following questions:

SPSS Tip ——————————————

In SPSS/PC, a two-way analysis of variance is performed using the ANOVA program, as in the following example:

```
ANOVA VARIABLES=DV BY IV1 (1,2) IV2 (1,2)
   /STATISTICS=3.
```

The ANOVA command instructs the computer to perform an analysis of variance for the dependent variable DV. The two independent variables are IV1 and IV2, both of which have a minimum value of 1 and a maximum value of 2, as shown in parentheses. The STATISTICS=3 subcommand instructs the computer to print the means and absolute frequencies for each cell in the design.

a. How many 4-year-old Children in the sample were Hispanic boys? How many were African-American girls?
b. Which group of 4-year-old Children was tallest, on average? Which group was shortest, on average?
c. For the ANOVA, what was the mean square between for the BCRACE main effect? What was the mean square between for the BCGENDER main effect? What was the mean square for the interaction term?
d. What was the value of the F statistic for the two main effects? What were the degrees of freedom for the main effects?
e. What was the value of the F statistic for the interaction? What were the degrees of freedom for the interaction effect?
f. Which effects, if any, were statistically significant at or beyond the .05 level?

B. INDEPENDENT COMPUTER EXERCISES

Use the NLSY data set to perform independent analyses of the type described in Chapter 7 of the textbook. Some specific suggestions follow.

1. Identify (or create) a nominal-level variable in the NLSY data set that has three or more categories and that is of substantive interest to you. Using this categorical variable as your independent variable, develop null hypotheses about the mean values for three (or more) dependent variables that are of substantive interest to you and that are meaningful in terms of the independent variable. Use the computer to perform one-way analyses of variance to test the three null hypotheses. Which of the null hypotheses are accepted and which are rejected at the .05 level of significance? At the .01 level of significance? Assuming a .05 level of significance, state your conclusions based on the one-way ANOVA for the three hypotheses, as they might be written for a research report, and prepare a table summarizing the results.

2. For the ANOVAs performed for Exercise B.1, perform multiple comparison tests to determine the nature of the relationship between the independent and dependent variable (*if* the ANOVAs were statistically significant). Are there any dependent variables for which all groups are significantly different from all other groups?

3. Compute eta^2 for the three analyses performed in Exercise B.1. For which dependent variable is the value of eta^2 greatest?

4. Identify a second categorical variable that is of interest to you as an independent variable. Perform two-way ANOVAs using both independent variables with the three dependent variables from Exercise B.1.

C. EXERCISES IN READING COMPUTER PRINTOUTS

The exercises in this section are based on printouts from a longitudinal study of over 2000 teenage mothers. Use the printouts to answer the questions included in the exercises.

1. Figure 7–1 presents an SPSS/PC printout for a one-way analysis of variance that examined the relationship between age at first birth (AGE1BRTH) and welfare receipt during the mother's childhood (WELFKID). Welfare status as a child was defined as a variable with three categories: never received welfare (code 1), received welfare some of the time (code 2), and received welfare throughout childhood (code 3). The ANOVA tested the null hypothesis that the young mother's age at first birth was unrelated to childhood welfare receipt:

H_0: $\mu_{\text{AGE1BRTH for WELFKID(1)}} = \mu_{\text{AGE1BRTH for WELFKID(2)}} = \mu_{\text{AGE1BRTH for WELFKID(3)}}$

Use the printout in Figure 7–1 to answer the following questions:

```
- - - - - - - - - - O N E W A Y - - - - - - - - - -
      Variable  AGE1BRTH    AGE WHEN 1ST GAVE BIRTH
   By Variable  WELFKID     RECVD WELFARE WHILE A CHILD?

                            Analysis of Variance
                            Sum of        Mean            F       F
          Source     D.F.   Squares       Squares      Ratio   Prob.

Between Groups        2      56.3369       28.1685     14.7598   .0000

Within Groups      2071    3952.4148        1.9085

Total              2073    4008.7517
```

Group	Count	Mean	Standard Deviation	Standard Error	95 Pct Conf Int for Mean		
NEVER	749	17.5251	1.3236	.0484	17.4301	To	17.6200
SOMETIME	980	17.2524	1.3972	.0446	17.1648	To	17.3400
ALWAYS	345	17.0770	1.4575	.0785	16.9227	To	17.2314
Total	2074	17.3217	1.3906	.0305	17.2618	To	17.3816

Group	Minimum	Maximum
NEVER	13.1253	20.7392
SOMETIME	10.0342	20.9774
ALWAYS	13.5305	20.9555.
Total	10.0342	20.9774

Levene Test for Homogeneity of Variances

Statistic	df1	df2	2-tail Sig.
2.2411	2	2071	.107

FIGURE 7–1. SPSS/PC PRINTOUT FOR EXERCISE C.1

a. How many young women in the sample never received welfare as a child? How many received welfare always as a child?

b. What are the mean ages at first birth for women in the three groups?

c. What is the mean square between groups and the mean square within groups in this ANOVA?

d. What is the value of the F statistic? What are the degrees of freedom?

e. At the .05 level of significance for a two-tailed test, can the null hypotheses be rejected? What is the exact probability level?

f. What is the 95% confidence level for the "never on welfare" group? Is there any overlap in the confidence intervals for the "never" group and the "always" group?

g. The Levene test was used to test the null hypothesis that the variances for the three populations are homogeneous. Should the null hypothesis be accepted or rejected?

h. Compute the value of eta^2, describing the magnitude of the relationship between age at first birth and childhood welfare receipt.

2. Figure 7–2 presents an SPSS/PC printout for a multiple comparison procedure (Fisher's LSD test) for the ANOVA shown in Figure 7–1. This procedure tests the following null hypotheses:

H_0: $\mu_{\text{AGE1BRTH for WELFKID(1)}} = \mu_{\text{AGE1BRTH for WELFKID(2)}}$

H_0: $\mu_{\text{AGE1BRTH for WELFKID(1)}} = \mu_{\text{AGE1BRTH for WELFKID(3)}}$

H_0: $\mu_{\text{AGE1BRTH for WELFKID(2)}} = \mu_{\text{AGE1BRTH for WELFKID(3)}}$

Use the printout in Figure 7–2 to answer the following questions:

a. What is the difference in mean age at first birth between the "never" group and the "sometimes" group?

b. Which groups are significantly different from one another with respect to age at first birth; i.e., which of the three null hypotheses can be rejected?

c. Assuming a .05 level of significance, state your conclusion based on the ANOVA and LSD test, as it might be written for a research report.

3. Figure 7–3 presents an SPSS/PC printout for a two-way ANOVA in which AGE1BRTH is once again the dependent variable. The two independent variables are welfare status as a child (WELFKID) and a dichotomous variable (AFR_AMER) indicating whether the mother is African-American (code 1) or not African-American (code 0). Use the printout in Figure 7–3 to answer the following questions:

a. How many African-American women were never on welfare as a child? How many non-African-American women were always on welfare as a child? How many missing cases were there in this analysis?

```
- - - - - - - - - - O N E W A Y - - - - - - - - - -
        Variable  AGE1BRTH   AGE WHEN 1ST GAVE BIRTH
     By Variable  WELFKID    RECVD WELFARE WHILE A CHILD?


Multiple Range Test


LSD Procedure
Ranges for the   .050 level -

        2.77    2.77

The ranges above are table ranges.
The value actually compared with Mean(J)-Mean(I) is..
        .9768 * Range * Sqrt(1/N(I) + 1/N(J))


(*) Denotes pairs of groups significantly different at the  .050 level

                              A S N
                              L O E
                              W M V
                              A E E
                              Y T R
                              S I
                                M
        Mean       Group      E

        17.0770    ALWAYS
        17.2524    SOMETIME   *
        17.5251    NEVER      * *
```

FIGURE 7–2. SPSS/PC PRINTOUT FOR EXERCISE C.2

b. Which group had the highest mean age at first birth and what was that mean? Which group had the lowest mean age at first birth and what was that mean?

c. What were the values of the F statistics for the two main effects? Which, if either, of the two main effects were statistically significant at or beyond the .05 level?

d. What was the value of the F statistic for the interaction effect? Was this effect statistically significant at or beyond the .05 level? Graph the means for the two independent variables to see more clearly what the interaction means.

4. Figure 7–4 presents a portion of an SPSS/PC printout for a mixed design repeated measures ANOVA in which the dependent variable is scores on the CES-D depression scale. The within-subjects factor is named TIMEFRAM—i.e., the time at which the scale was administered (at the baseline interview—BASECESD—or at the 18-month follow-up interview—CESD). The between-subjects factor is welfare status as a child (WELFKID), as defined in the previous exercises. Panel A of the printout presents basic

```
* * *   C E L L   M E A N S   * * *

        AGE1BRTH  AGE WHEN 1ST GAVE BIRTH
     BY WELFKID   RECVD WELFARE WHILE A CHILD?
        AFR_AMER


        AFR_AMER
                 0            1
WELFKID
     1      17.68       17.32
         (   428)   (    321)

     2      17.52       17.05
         (   424)   (    556)

     3      17.05       17.09
         (   135)   (    210)
```

```
* * *   A N A L Y S I S   O F   V A R I A N C E   * * *

        AGE1BRTH  AGE WHEN 1ST GAVE BIRTH
     BY   WELFKID  RECVD WELFARE WHILE A CHILD?
          AFR_AMER
```

Source of Variation	Sum of Squares	DF	Mean Square	F	Signif of F
Main Effects	117.552	3	39.184	20.912	.000
WELFKID	39.721	2	19.860	10.599	.000
AFR_AMER	61.215	1	61.215	32.670	.000
2-way Interactions	16.255	2	8.127	4.338	.013
WELFKID AFR_AMER	16.255	2	8.127	4.338	.013
Explained	133.807	5	26.761	14.282	.000
Residual	3874.944	2068	1.874		
Total	4008.752	2073	1.934		

```
2106 Cases were processed.
  32 Cases (  1.5 PCT) were missing.
```

FIGURE 7–3. SPSS/PC PRINTOUT FOR EXERCISE C.3

descriptive statistics, Panel B shows the ANOVA results for the between-subjects factor, and Panel C shows the ANOVA results for the within-subjects factor and the interaction. Use Figure 7–4 to answer the following questions:

a. What was the mean depression scale score at baseline for women never on welfare as a child? What was the mean depression scale score at follow-up for women always on welfare as a child?

A Cell Means and Standard Deviations
Variable .. BASECESD   DEPRESSION SCORE AT BASELINE
        FACTOR   CODE   Mean Std. Dev.   N

    WELFKID   NEVER   17.296   10.274   749
    WELFKID   SOMETIME   18.182   10.104   978
    WELFKID   ALWAYS   19.690   10.522   345
For entire sample   18.113   10.263   2072

- - - - - - - - -

Variable .. CESD   DEPRESSION SCORE 1ST FOLLOWUP
        FACTOR   CODE   Mean Std. Dev.   N

    WELFKID   NEVER   15.406   10.535   749
    WELFKID   SOMETIME   16.153   10.322   978
    WELFKID   ALWAYS   16.855   10.784   345
For entire sample   16.000   10.484   2072

B * * ANALYSIS OF VARIANCE -- DESIGN   1 * *

Tests of Between-Subjects Effects.

Tests of Significance for T1 using UNIQUE sums of squares
Source of Variation   SS   DF   MS   F Sig of F

WITHIN CELLS   314898.08   2069   152.20
CONSTANT   1020645.47   1 1020645.5   6706.03   .000
WELFKID   1789.71   2   894.85   5.88   .003

C Tests involving 'TIMEFRAM' Within-Subject Effect.

Tests of Significance for T2 using UNIQUE sums of squares
Source of Variation   SS   DF   MS   F Sig of F

WITHIN CELLS   128991.90   2069   62.35
TIMEFRAM   4339.25   1   4339.25   69.60   .000
WELFKID BY TIMEFRAM   111.88   2   55.94   .90   .408

FIGURE 7–4. SPSS/PC PRINTOUT FOR EXERCISE C.4

b. For which group did level of depression improve the most, on average?
c. Were depression scale scores significantly related to welfare status as a child, at the .05 level? What was the value of the F statistic for the between-subjects factor?
d. Did depression scale scores change significantly over time, at the .05 level? What was the value of the F statistic for the within-subjects factor?
e. Was the interaction between the between-subjects and within-subjects factors significant at the .05 level? What was the value of the F statistic for the interaction term?

Chi-Square and
Other Nonparametric Tests

A. DIRECTED COMPUTER EXERCISES

Appendixes A, B, and C of this Manual list all the variables in the NLSY data set contained on the enclosed diskette. Perform the analyses described in the following exercises using the NLSY data set, and then answer the accompanying questions.

1. Test the null hypothesis that the focal Child's race/ethnicity (BCRACE) is unrelated to whether or not he or she was breastfed (HLBRFED) as an infant, using a chi-square test. Also generate information on the value of Cramér's V.

Use the printout to answer the following questions:

a. How many Hispanic Children were breastfed? What percentage of African-American Children were breastfed? What percentage of the sample were *not* breastfed?
b. What is the absolute frequency of non-Hispanic, non-African-American Children who were breastfed? What is the *expected* frequency for this group?
c. What is the value of the chi-square statistic? How many degrees of freedom are there?
d. Can the null hypothesis be rejected, based on conventional levels of statistical significance? What is the probability that the Child's race/ethnicity and breastfeeding history are independent?
e. Assuming a .05 level of significance, state your conclusion based on the chi-square test, as it might be written for a research report.

SPSS Tip ──────────────────────────

In SPSS/PC, a chi-square test is performed using the CROSSTABS command, as in the following example:

CROSSTABS TABLES=DV BY IV
  /CELLS=COUNT COLUMN TOTAL EXPECTED
  /STATISTICS=CHISQ PHI.

As explained in Chapter 4, the CROSSTABS program crosstabulates the variables specified after TABLES=; here, DV is crosstabulated by IV. The CELLS= subcommand tells the computer what information is to be presented in each cell of the contingency table; in this case, each cell will show the absolute frequency, column percentage, total percentage, and the expected frequency. The STATISTICS=CHISQ PHI subcommand indicates that a chi-square test is to be performed, and that phi/Cramér's V is to be computed.

───

    2. Test the hypothesis that the month in which prenatal care during the mother's pregnancy with the focal Child began (PRMOCARE) is unrelated to whether the mother was living in poverty (BMPOVERT, coded 1 if in poverty and 0 if not in poverty), using the Mann-Whitney U-test.
    When you have produced the printout, use it to answer the following questions:

a. How many women were living in poverty? How many were not?
b. What is the value of the U statistic? What is the corresponding value of Z (the statistic for the Wilcoxon rank sum test)?
c. Can the null hypothesis be rejected at conventional levels of statistical significance? What is the probability that the population distributions for the prenatal care variable are identical in the two poverty status groups?
d. Assuming a .05 level of significance, state your conclusion based on the Mann-Whitney U-test, as it might be written for a research report.

    3. Test the null hypothesis that the mother's self-rating of shyness (BMSHY85) is unrelated to her marital status (BMMARST), using the Kruskal-Wallis test.
    When you have produced the printout, use it to answer the following questions:

SPSS Tip

In SPSS/PC, over a dozen nonparametric tests can be run within the program NPAR TESTS. The following is an example of the commands for the Mann-Whitney U-test:

NPAR TESTS M-W=DV BY IV (1,2).

The designation M-W after NPAR TESTS indicates that the test to be performed is the Mann-Whitney. A dependent variable named DV will be tested in relation to an independent variable named IV, whose categories are coded 1 and 2.

---

a. How many women were never married? How many were neither currently married nor never married (i.e., were separated, divorced or widowed)?
b. What is the value of the test statistic (chi-square or H)?
c. Can the null hypothesis be rejected at conventional levels of statistical significance? What is the probability that the population distributions for the shyness ratings are identical in the three marital status groups?
d. Assuming a .05 level of significance, state your conclusion based on the Kruskal-Wallis test, as it might be written for a research report.

SPSS Tip

In SPSS/PC, the program NPAR TESTS is used for the Kruskal-Wallis test, as in the following example:

NPAR TESTS K-W=DV BY IV (1,4).

The designation K-W after NPAR TESTS indicates that the test to be performed is the Kruskal-Wallis. A dependent variable named DV is to be tested in relation to an independent variable named IV, whose categories are coded from 1 to 4.

B. INDEPENDENT COMPUTER EXERCISES

Use the NLSY data set to perform independent analyses of the type described in Chapter 8 of the textbook. Some specific suggestions follow.

1. Identify five nominal-level variables in the NLSY data set that are of substantive interest to you. Crosstabulate them all by another nominal-level variable of interest to you. Perform a chi-square test of independence to determine the relationship between the variables. Also compute phi or Cramér's V. Select one of the tests (preferably one with nonsignificant results) and use the results as the basis for a power analysis. How many subjects would be needed to achieve a power of .80 with an alpha of .05?

2. Identify an ordinal-level variable in the NLSY data set that is of substantive interest to you. Use the computer to test the relationship between this variable and the Child's gender (or another nominal-level variable of interest to you), using either the Mann-Whitney U-test or the Kruskal-Wallis test, as appropriate.

C. EXERCISES IN READING COMPUTER PRINTOUTS

The exercises in this section are based on printouts from a longitudinal study of over 2000 teenage mothers. Use the printouts to answer the questions included in the exercises.

1. Figure 8-1 presents an SPSS/PC printout of a contingency table that crosstabulated two dichotomous variables: whether the mother had used any drugs (marijuana, cocaine, crack, PCP, etc.) in the previous month (ANYDRUG, coded 0 if no, 1 if yes) and whether the mother had been hospitalized at any time since the baseline interview, other than for childbirth (HOSPITAL, coded 1 if yes, 2 if no). A chi-square test of independence was performed and the phi statistic was computed. Using the printout in Figure 8-1, answer the following questions:

a. State the null hypothesis being tested.
b. How many young mothers had been hospitalized since baseline? What percentage of the sample with valid data was this?
c. How many young mothers had used drugs in the past month? What percentage of the sample with valid data was this?
d. Among the mothers who used drugs, what percentage had been hospitalized? How much higher was this than the percentage who had not used drugs?
e. What was the value of chi-square (χ^2)? What was the value of chi-square after Yates' correction?
f. Based on the chi-square test, can the null hypothesis be rejected at conventional levels of statistical significance? What is the probability that the mother's drug use is independent of her hospitalization record since baseline?
g. What is the value of the phi statistic?
h. Assuming a .05 level of significance, state your conclusion based on the chi-square test, as it might be written for a research report.

```
HOSPITAL  IN HOSPITAL SINCE BASELINE?  by  ANYDRUG  USED ANY DRUG PAST MONTH?

                      ANYDRUG        Page 1 of 1
                Count
                Exp Val |NO DRUGS USED DRU
                Col Pct | PAST MO GS PAST   Row
                        |    .00|    1.00| Total
HOSPITAL        --------+--------+--------+
        1.00    |    127 |     30 |    157
  YES           |  133.7 |   23.3 |  15.1%
                |  14.3% |  19.4% |
                +--------+--------+
        2.00    |    761 |    125 |    886
   NO           |  754.3 |  131.7 |  84.9%
                |  85.7% |  80.6% |
                +--------+--------+
        Column       888      155     1043
        Total      85.1%    14.9%   100.0%
```

Chi-Square	Value	DF	Significance
Pearson	2.63512	1	.10452
Continuity Correction	2.25476	1	.13320
Likelihood Ratio	2.48713	1	.11478
Mantel-Haenszel test for linear association	2.63259	1	.10469

Minimum Expected Frequency -   23.332

Statistic	Value	ASE1	T-value	Approximate Significance
Phi	.05026			.10452 *1
Cramer's V	.05026			.10452 *1

FIGURE 8-1. SPSS/PC PRINTOUT FOR EXERCISE C.1

2. Figure 8–2 presents an SPSS/PC printout of a Kruskal-Wallis test in which the mother's number of sick days since baseline (SICKDAYS) is the dependent variable and her clinical depression category is the independent variable (DEPRESS, coded 0 if not at risk of clinical depression, 1 if at risk, and 2 if at high risk). Use the printout to answer the following questions:

a. What is the null hypothesis being tested?
b. Which group had the highest mean rank for the SICKDAYS variable? How many cases were in this group?
c. What is the value of the chi-square statistic, before and after correction for ties?
d. Based on the Kruskal-Wallis test, can the null hypothesis be rejected at conventional levels of statistical significance? What is the probability that at-risk status is unrelated to number of sick days since baseline?
e. Assuming a .05 level of significance, state your conclusion based on the Kruskal-Wallis test, as it might be written for a research report.

```
- - - - - Kruskal-Wallis 1-way ANOVA

      SICKDAYS   # SICK DAYS SINCE BASELINE
   by DEPRESS    AT RISK OF CLINICL DEPRESSN-FRM CESD SCA


      Mean Rank     Cases

         495.74        627    DEPRESS = 0    NOT AT RISK
         531.88        211    DEPRESS = 1    AT RISK
         585.48        202    DEPRESS = 2    AT HIGH RISK
                       ----
                      1040    Total

                                                 Corrected for Ties
         CASES    Chi-Square  Significance   Chi-Square  Significance
         1040      14.0182         .0009      15.3982         .0005
```

FIGURE 8–2. SPSS/PC PRINTOUT FOR EXERCISE C.2

3. Figure 8–3 presents an SPSS/PC printout of a Wilcoxon signed-ranks test. One variable measures the mother's frequency of using marijuana in the previous month (MARUSE) and the other measures the mother's frequency of using cocaine in the previous month (COCUSE). Use the printout to answer the following questions:

a. What is the null hypothesis being tested?
b. For how many cases was the frequency of marijuana use the same as the frequency of cocaine use? For how many cases was the frequency of marijuana use greater than the frequency of cocaine use?
c. What is the value of the Z statistic?
d. Based on the Wilcoxon signed-ranks test, can the null hypothesis be rejected at conventional levels of statistical significance? What is the probability value?
e. Assuming a .05 level of significance, state your conclusion based on the Wilcoxon signed-ranks test, as it might be written for a research report.

```
- - - - - Wilcoxon Matched-pairs Signed-ranks Test

      MARUSE     FREQ OF MARIJUANA USE PAST MO
   with COCUSE   FREQ OF COCAINE USE PAST MO


      Mean Rank     Cases

         137.58        262    - Ranks (COCUSE Lt MARUSE)
         135.67         12    + Ranks (COCUSE Gt MARUSE)
                      1813    Ties  (COCUSE Eq MARUSE)
                      ----
                      2087    Total

         Z = -13.1083              2-tailed P = .0000
```

FIGURE 8–3. SPSS/PC PRINTOUT FOR EXERCISE C.3

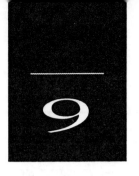

9

Correlation and Simple Regression

A. DIRECTED COMPUTER EXERCISES

Appendixes A, B, and C of this Manual list all the variables in the NLSY data set contained on the enclosed diskette. Perform the analyses described in the following exercises using the NLSY data set, and then answer the accompanying questions.

    1. The variable BMAGEMEN indicates the age at which the focal Child's mother began menstruation and BMAGEINT indicates the age at which the mother first had sexual intercourse. Test the null hypothesis that these two variables are uncorrelated (i.e., H_0: = .00). At the same time, generate basic descriptive statistics (mean, *SD*) for the two variables.

    When you have produced the printout, use it to answer the following questions:

a. What was the mean age at which the mothers reached menarche? What was their mean age at first intercourse?
b. What is the correlation between the two variables?
c. At the .05 level, is the correlation between the two variables statistically significant? What is the actual probability that the null hypothesis is true?
d. Write a sentence describing the results of the hypothesis test.

    2. Use the computer to generate a correlation matrix for the following variables: PRWTGAIN (number of pounds the mother gained during her pregnancy with the focal Child), PRBWT (the Child's birth weight); PRBLENG (the Child's length at birth), PRMHOSP (number of days the mother was in the hospital at the Child's birth), and PRCHOSP (number of days the Child was in the hospital at birth). Use *listwise* deletion of missing cases (see Chapter 4). When you have produced the printout, use the matrix to answer the following questions:

SPSS Tip ─────────────────────────────────

In SPSS/PC, descriptive statistics can be generated at the same time as Pearson's r using the STATISTICS subcommand of the CORRELATIONS program, as in this example:

CORRELATIONS VARIABLES=DV, IV
    /STATISTICS=1.

This command will correlate the two variables specified (DV and IV) and will also yield information on their means, SDs, and frequencies.

───

a. Which two variables in the matrix are *most* strongly correlated? What is the value of Pearson's r for that correlation? Is the correlation significant at the .05 level? What is the probability that the variables are unrelated in the population?
b. Which two variables in the matrix are *least* strongly correlated? What is the value of Pearson's r for that correlation? Is the correlation significant at the .05 level? What is the probability that the variables are unrelated in the population?
c. Write a sentence describing the results of the tests of the null hypotheses that the Child's birth weight is unrelated to (1) his or her length of stay in the hospital and (2) the mother's stay in the hospital.

     3. Test the hypothesis that the relationship between maternal weight gain during pregnancy and the baby's length at birth is zero—*separately for male and female infants.* (In other words, compute the correlation coefficient between PRWTGAIN and PRBLENG separately for the two different values of BCGENDER.) When you have produced the printout, use it to answer the following questions:

a. What is the value of Pearson's r for the male infants? Is the correlation significant at the .05 level? What is the probability that the variables are unrelated in the population?
b. What is the value of Pearson's r for the female infants? Is the correlation significant at the .05 level? What is the probability that the variables are unrelated in the population?
c. Transform each of the two rs to values of z, using the r-to-z transformation table in Appendix B of the textbook (Table B–7). What are the z values?
d. Test the hypothesis that the relationship between PRWTGAIN and PRBLENG is equivalent for male and female infants. What is the value of z_{obs}? Are the two correlations significantly different at the .05 level?

SPSS Tip

In SPSS/PC, one approach to computing Spearman's r_S is to use the CROSSTABS program, as in the following example:

```
CROSSTABS TABLES=DV BY IV
  /FORMAT=NOTABLES
  /STATISTICS=CORR.
```

The STATISTICS=CORR subcommand will generate both Spearman's r_S and Pearson's r between the named variables (here, DV and IV). The FORMAT=NOTABLES subcommand ensures that the crosstabulation table is not printed.

---

4. Two variables in the NLSY data set that are measured on an ordinal scale are BCFADIST (the distance between the focal Child's residence and his or her father's residence) and BCSEEFA (the frequency with which the Child sees the father). Use Spearman's rank-order correlation to test the hypothesis that these two variables are unrelated.

When you have produced the printout, use it to answer the following questions:

a. What is the value of Spearman's r_S between BCFADIST and BCSEEFA?
b. Is the correlation significant at the .05 level? What is the probability that the variables are unrelated in the population?
c. Write a sentence describing the results of the hypothesis test.

SPSS Tip

In SPSS/PC, linear regression can be performed using the REGRESSION procedure, as in the following example:

```
REGRESSION VARIABLES=DV IV
  /DEPENDENT=DV
  /METHOD=ENTER IV.
```

These commands indicate that the variables in the regression are DV and IV, and that the dependent variable is DV. The subcommand METHOD=ENTER tells the computer to regress DV on IV.

5. Use the computer to regress the focal Child's birth weight (PRBWT) on the mother's weight gain during her pregnancy (PRWTGAIN), i.e., to predict the Child's birth weight on the basis of maternal weight gain.

When you have produced the printout, use it to answer the following questions:

a. What is the value of r? What is the value of r^2?
b. What is the standard error of estimate for predicting values of the Child's birth weight?
c. What is the regression equation?

B. INDEPENDENT COMPUTER EXERCISES

Use the NLSY data set to perform independent analyses of the type described in Chapter 9 of the textbook. Some specific suggestions follow.

1. Develop a hypothesis involving the relationship between two variables in the NLSY data set measured on the interval or ratio scale. Use correlational procedures to test the hypothesis.

2. Using the computer, compute the correlation between two variables in the NLSY data set, separately for two distinct subgroups (e.g., males versus females, African-Americans versus non-African-Americans, low-birth-weight infants versus normal- birth-weight infants, etc.). Test the hypothesis that the correlations for the two subgroups are equivalent.

3. Using linear regression, develop a prediction equation to predict one variable in the NLSY data set (Y) based on a second variable (X) that you believe would be a good predictor. Then use a listing procedure (see Chapter 1) to list the *actual* values of X and Y for the first five cases in the file. Manually compute Y for these five cases, based on actual values of X and the regression equation. Examine the accuracy of the prediction by comparing Y and Y'.

C. EXERCISES IN READING COMPUTER PRINTOUTS

The exercises in this section are based on printouts from a longitudinal study of over 2000 teenage mothers. Use the printouts to answer the questions included in the exercises.

1. Figure 9–1 presents a printout with a correlation matrix for four variables, each of which corresponded to an aspect of the young mothers' parenting attitudes:

ANGRY   I often feel angry with my child.
TRAPPED   I feel trapped by my responsibilities as a parent.
NOTCRY   I think children must learn early not to cry.
HARDKID   My child seems to be much harder to care for than most.

The young mothers responded to each statement on a 0 to 10 scale, where 0 meant "not at all true" and 10 meant "completely true." Use the printout to answer the following questions:

Variable	Cases	Mean	Std Dev
TRAPPED	2013	2.5648	3.0948
ANGRY	2013	2.3686	2.5705
NOTCRY	2013	2.3000	3.0263
HARDKID	2013	1.9344	2.5066

Correlations:	TRAPPED	ANGRY	NOTCRY	HARDKID
TRAPPED	1.0000 (2013) P= .	.2645 (2013) P= .000	.1049 (2013) P= .000	.2700 (2013) P= .000
ANGRY	.2645 (2013) P= .000	1.0000 (2013) P= .	.1515 (2013) P= .000	.2372 (2013) P= .000
NOTCRY	.1049 (2013) P= .000	.1515 (2013) P= .000	1.0000 (2013) P= .	.1290 (2013) P= .000
HARDKID	.2700 (2013) P= .000	.2372 (2013) P= .000	.1290 (2013) P= .000	1.0000 (2013) P= .

(Coefficient / (Cases) / 2-tailed Significance)

" . " is printed if a coefficient cannot be computed

FIGURE 9–1. SPSS/PC PRINTOUT FOR EXERCISE C.1

a. Which variable has the greatest variability of responses?
b. Which variable has the lowest mean (i.e., lowest average level of endorsement)?
c. Which two variables have the highest correlation? What was the value of r?
d. Which two variables have the lowest correlation? What was the value of r?
e. Are there correlations that are not statistically significant at or beyond the .05 level? If so, for which variable pairs are the correlations not significant?

2. Figure 9–2 presents a printout for a linear regression. The two variables in the analysis are:

HOME@TOT Score on the Home Observation for Measurement of the Environment (HOME) Scale, a scale that measures the quality of the focal Child's home environment
NKIDS The number of children of the young mother

Use the printout to answer the following questions:

```
* * * *   M U L T I P L E   R E G R E S S I O N   * * * *
```

Listwise Deletion of Missing Data

```
              Mean    Std Dev   Label

HOME@TOT   100.535     14.990   HOME ENVIRONMT SCALE TOTAL SCORE
NKIDS        1.691       .819   NUMBER OF CHILDREN
```

N of Cases = 1965

Correlation:

```
            HOME@TOT        NKIDS

HOME@TOT     1.000         -.215
NKIDS        -.215          1.000
```

Equation Number 1   Dependent Variable..   HOME@TOT   HOME ENVIRONMT SCALE TOT

Block Number 1. Method: Enter   NKIDS

Variable(s) Entered on Step Number
    1..   NKIDS   NUMBER OF CHILDREN

```
Multiple R           .21511
R Square             .04627
Adjusted R Square    .04579
Standard Error     14.64272
```

Analysis of Variance

```
                   DF    Sum of Squares    Mean Square
Regression          1       20419.85178    20419.85178
Residual         1963      420885.21207      214.40918
```

F =   95.23777   Signif F = .0000

------------------ Variables in the Equation -------------------

```
Variable              B        SE B       Beta         T    Sig T

NKIDS          -3.936308     .403352    -.215108    -9.759   .0000
(Constant)    107.189231     .757696                141.467   .0000
```

End Block Number   1   All requested variables entered.

FIGURE 9–2. SPSS/PC PRINTOUT FOR EXERCISE C.2

a. What is the mean HOME score? What is the *SD*? What do these values suggest?
b. In the regression analysis, which is the dependent variable (*Y*) and which is the predictor variable (*X*)?
c. What is the correlation between the two variables? What is the value of r^2?
d. What is the prediction equation?
e. What would be the predicted HOME score for a woman with four children?

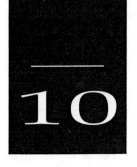

Multiple Regression

A. DIRECTED COMPUTER EXERCISES

Appendixes A, B, and C of this Manual list all the variables in the NLSY data set contained on the enclosed diskette. Perform the analyses described in the following exercises using the NLSY data set, and then answer the accompanying questions.

1. Use multiple regression to predict the focal Child's birth weight (PRBWT) based on maternal weight gain during pregnancy (PRWTGAIN) *and* mother's prepregnancy weight (PRWTBEF), using the simultaneous regression approach.

When you have produced the printout, use it to answer the following questions:

a. What is the multiple correlation between the dependent variable and the predictors? What is R^2 (unadjusted and adjusted)?
b. What is the standard error of estimate? In what units is this value?
c. What is the value of F for the overall regression? Is this F statistically significant at conventional levels? What is the probability that the multiple correlation coefficient in the population is zero?
d. Which (if either) of the two predictors is statistically significant? At what probability level?
e. What is the multiple regression equation for predicting PRBWT (Y') from PRWTGAIN (X_1) and PRWTBEF (X_2)?
f. For those who completed Exercise A.5 of Chapter 9 (the simple regression of PRBWT on PRWTGAIN), what is the increment to R^2 by adding PRWTBEF to the prediction equation?

SPSS Tip ―――――――――――――――――――――――

In SPSS/PC, multiple regression is performed using the REGRESSION procedure. The REGRESSION program is complex and offers the analyst numerous options, a full description of which is provided in the SPSS manual. A basic simultaneous regression can be produced using the following commands:

REGRESSION VARIABLES=IV1 IV2 DV
  /DEPENDENT=DV
  /METHOD=ENTER
  /DESCRIPTIVES.

These commands indicate that the variables in the regression are IV1, IV2, and DV, and that the dependent variable is DV. The subcommand METHOD=ENTER tells the computer to regress DV on all other variables specified after the VARIABLES= keyword simultaneously (i.e., on IV1 and IV2 in this example). The DESCRIPTIVES subcommand generates means, SDs, and other descriptive statistics for all variables in the equation.

――

2. Perform a hierarchical regression to predict the focal Child's birth weight (PRBWT); that is, after first holding PRWTGAIN and PRWTBEF constant, add the mother's age at first birth (BMAGE1ST) to the regression equation in a second step. Test the tolerance to ensure there are no multicollinearity problems.

When you have produced the printout, use it to answer the following questions:

a. What is the multiple correlation between PRBWT and the *three* predictor variables? What is the value of R^2?
b. What is the *change* in R^2 when BMAGE1ST is entered into the equation? Is this change statistically significant at conventional levels? What is the value of F for the change?
c. Does the value of F for the *overall* equation increase, decrease, or stay the same when BMAGE1ST is added to the regression?
d. Are the tolerance levels acceptable for the three variables in the equation; i.e., is there evidence of multicollinearity?
e. What is the multiple regression equation *in standardized form* for predicting PRBWT (z_Y) from PRWTGAIN (z_{X_1}), PRWTBEF (z_{X_2}), and BMAGE1ST (z_{X_3})?

SPSS Tip

In SPSS/PC, the REGRESSION program allows the entry of variables in consecutive steps through multiple METHOD=ENTER commands, as in the following example:

```
REGRESSION VARIABLES=IV1 IV2 IV3 IV4 DV
  /STATISTICS=DEFAULTS CHA TOL
  /DEPENDENT=DV
  /METHOD=ENTER IV1 IV2
  /METHOD=ENTER IV3 IV4
  /DESCRIPTIVES.
```

These commands specify that the dependent variable is DV. The first METHOD=ENTER subcommand instructs the computer to enter the predictors IV1 and IV2 into the regression equation simultaneously. Then, the second METHOD=ENTER subcommand instructs the computer to add IV3 and IV4 into the equation in a subsequent step. The STATISTICS subcommand (placed directly before the specification of the dependent variable) requests the DEFAULTS (R, the overall F statistic) plus CHA (the change in R^2 for any step after the first) and TOL (tolerance level). (The STATISTICS subcommand does not need to be included if *only* the default statistics are desired.)

---

3. The variable PRSMOKE in the NLSY data set indicates how much the mother smoked during her pregnancy with the focal Child. As currently coded, the variable cannot be used in multiple regression because it is an ordinal-level variable. Create a dummy variable (call it NOSMOKE) that could be used as a predictor in multiple regression, contrasting those who never smoked during their pregnancies (code 1) and those who did smoke. Use the computer to calculate the mean and *SD* for the dummy variable.

4. Use stepwise regression to predict PRBWT on the basis of PRWTGAIN, PRWTBEF, BMAGE1ST, and NOSMOKE. Use .05 as the minimum probability value for entering variables into the equation.

When you have produced the printout, use it to answer the following questions:

a. What is the first variable stepped into the regression equation? What is the value of R^2 at that point?

SPSS Tip ————————————————————————————————

In SPSS/PC, dummy coding can be achieved through COMPUTE and IF commands or through recoding of variables. As an example, suppose we wanted to use the variable BCRACE (the focal Child's race/ethnicity) to create a dummy variable to contrast Hispanic children and all other Children. The following commands could be used:

COMPUTE HISPANIC=0.
IF (BCRACE EQ 1) HISPANIC=1.

The first command sets the new variable (HISPANIC) equal to 0 for all cases. The second command sets the new variable equal to 1 if and only if the Child is Hispanic, i.e., if the case has a code of 1 (Hispanic) for the original variable BCRACE.

SPSS Tip ————————————————————————————————

In SPSS/PC, the REGRESSION program can be instructed to perform a stepwise regression through the METHOD subcommand, as in the following example:

REGRESSION VARIABLES=IV1 IV2 IV3 DV
  /CRITERIA=PIN (.01)
  /STATISTICS=DEFAULTS CHA TOL
  /DEPENDENT=DV
  /METHOD=STEPWISE
  /DESCRIPTIVES.

These commands specify that the dependent variable is DV and that all other variables on the VARIABLES= list (IV1 to IV3) are the predictors that are to be entered by the stepwise method (METHOD=STEPWISE). In SPSS, the default probability level to enter variables in or out is .05, and therefore the CRITERIA subcommand often can be omitted. In this example, variables are stepped into the equation only if the probability for the entering variable is .01 or lower.

b. What is the second variable stepped into the regression equation? How much does R^2 change? Is the second predictor the variable with the second highest bivariate correlation with PRBWT?

c. After the second step, are there any remaining variables whose p value meets the .05 criterion for variable entry? If yes, which variable is that?

d. Are there any variables that do *not* meet the .05 criterion for variable entry? If yes, which are the variables and what are the associated p levels?

e. What is the final value of R^2?

B. INDEPENDENT COMPUTER EXERCISES

Use the NLSY data set to perform independent analyses of the type described in Chapter 10 of the textbook. Some specific suggestions follow.

1. Develop a hypothesis for a three-variable multiple regression analysis. That is, select an interval-level or ratio-level variable in the NLSY data set that you would like to predict or explain (Y) and then select two variables (X_1 and X_2) that you believe would be good predictors. Use simultaneous regression to enter the predictor variables.

2. Using a hierarchical approach, add one more variable—a nominal-level variable with at least three categories—that you believe would significantly improve the predictive ability of the equation specified in Exercise B.1. First use dummy coding, and then use effect coding to represent the nominal-level variable. Compare the values of the intercept and the regression coefficients for the two coding methods.

3. Use stepwise regression to predict the Y variable from Exercises B.1 and B.2 based on all predictors used thus far. Are all the independent variables significant predictors of Y?

4. Inspect the output from the regression analyses in the previous three exercises for any evidence of suppression.

C. EXERCISES IN READING COMPUTER PRINTOUTS

The exercises in this section are based on printouts from a longitudinal study of over 2000 teenage mothers. Use the printouts to answer the questions included in the exercises.

1. Figure 10–1 presents a printout for a simultaneous multiple regression. The three variables in the analysis are:

HOME@TOT   Score on the Home Observation for Measurement of the Environment (HOME) Scale, a scale that measures the quality of the focal Child's home environment

NKIDS   The number of children of the young mother
CESD   Mother's score on the CES-D depression scale

The dependent variable in the analysis is HOME@TOT. Use the printout to answer the following questions:

a. What is the multiple correlation between HOME@TOT and the two predictors? What is R^2 (unadjusted and adjusted)? Why is the adjusted value so similar to the unadjusted value?

b. What is the value of F for the overall regression? Is this F statistically significant at conventional levels? What is the probability that the multiple correlation coefficient in the population is zero? What are the degrees of freedom for the F test?

c. What is the value of the t statistic associated with CESD? Holding NKIDS constant, is CESD statistically significant? At what probability level?

```
* * * *    M U L T I P L E    R E G R E S S I O N    * * * *

Equation Number 1    Dependent Variable..    HOME@TOT    HOME ENVIRONMT SCALE TOT

Block Number  1.  Method:  Enter      NKIDS    CESD


Variable(s) Entered on Step Number
   1..    CESD       DEPRESSION SCORE 1ST FOLLOWUP
   2..    NKIDS      NUMBER OF CHILDREN


Multiple R           .28665
R Square             .08217
Adjusted R Square    .08123
Standard Error     14.36818

Analysis of Variance
                    DF      Sum of Squares      Mean Square
Regression           2         36260.58201      18130.29101
Residual          1962        405044.48183        206.44469

F =      87.82154      Signif F =  .0000


------------------ Variables in the Equation ------------------

Variable           B          SE B        Beta          T    Sig T

CESD          -.277301      .031657     -.189590     -8.760   .0000
NKIDS        -3.807806      .396062     -.208086     -9.614   .0000
(Constant)  111.359410      .882847                 126.137   .0000


End Block Number   1   All requested variables entered.
```

FIGURE 10–1. SPSS/PC PRINTOUT FOR EXERCISE C.1

d. State what the regression coefficient associated with CESD means.

e. What is the multiple regression equation for predicting HOME@TOT (Y) from CESD (X_1) and NKIDS (X_2)?

2. Figure 10–2 presents a portion of a printout for a stepwise multiple regression analysis in which HOME@TOT (see exercise C.1) is the dependent variable. The independent variables in the analysis are NKIDS and CESD, as in the previous exercise, plus the following variables:

HUSBAND   Whether the young mother is currently married and living with a husband (0 = no, 1 = yes)

ANYDRUG   Whether the young mother has used any drug in the previous month (0 = no, 1 = yes)

DIPLOMA   Whether the young mother has received her high school diploma (0 = no, 1 = yes)

Figure 10–2 shows the printout at the third step of the stepwise regression. Use the printout to answer the following questions:

a. What variable was entered on the third step? What was the change in R^2 for adding that variable? What was the F statistic associated with the change?

b. What variables were already in the equation at that point; i.e., what variables were entered on the first two steps?

c. Is having a husband associated with a predicted increase or decrease in HOME scores? How much of an increase/decrease, after controlling other variables already entered?

d. Using squared semipartial correlations (Part Cor), about how much more "important" a predictor of HOME scores is number of children than presence of a husband in the household?

e. What variables are not yet in the equation at the third step? Using a default criterion of .05 for entering predictors, would there be a fourth step? If so, what variable would enter on the fourth step?

f. Is multicollinearity a problem in this analysis?

* * * *   M U L T I P L E   R E G R E S S I O N   * * * *

Equation Number 2   Dependent Variable..   HOME@TOT   HOME ENVIRONMT SCALE TOT

Variable(s) Entered on Step Number
    3..   HUSBAND   HUSBAND OF R IN HH?

Multiple R	.30794		
R Square	.09482	R Square Change	.01266
Adjusted R Square	.09344	F Change	27.42315
Standard Error	14.27240	Signif F Change	.0000

Analysis of Variance

	DF	Sum of Squares	Mean Square
Regression	3	41846.71547	13948.90516
Residual	1961	399458.34838	203.70135

F =   68.47723   Signif F =   .0000

---------------------- Variables in the Equation ----------------------

Variable	B	SE B	Beta	Correl	Part Cor	Partial
NKIDS	-3.937073	.394195	-.215150	-.215108	-.214580	-.220014
CESD	-.268264	.031493	-.183412	-.197298	-.183011	-.188895
HUSBAND	6.332378	1.209228	.112885	.109471	.112509	.117437
(Constant)	110.945131	.880522				

----------- Variables in the Equation -----------

Variable	Tolerance	VIF	T	Sig T
NKIDS	.994712	1.005	-9.988	.0000
CESD	.995630	1.004	-8.518	.0000
HUSBAND	.993342	1.007	5.237	.0000
(Constant)			125.999	.0000

---------------------- Variables not in the Equation ----------------------

Variable	Beta In	Partial	Tolerance	VIF	Min Toler	T	Sig T
ANYDRUG	-.088211	-.091734	.978927	1.022	.978736	-4.078	.0000
DIPLOMA	.105664	.109066	.964413	1.037	.964413	4.858	.0000

FIGURE 10–2. SPSS/PC PRINTOUT FOR EXERCISE C.2

Analysis of Covariance, Multivariate ANOVA, and Canonical Analysis

A. DIRECTED COMPUTER EXERCISES

Appendixes A, B, and C of this Manual list all the variables in the NLSY data set contained on the enclosed diskette. Perform the analyses described in the following exercises using the NLSY data set, and then answer the accompanying questions.

 1. Are there differences among young women from different racial/ethnic groups with regard to desired family size (i.e., number of children)? Use analysis of covariance to test the null hypothesis that the three groups of mothers in the NLSY data set (Hispanics, African-Americans, and others, as defined by BCRACE[1]) did not have different family size desires in 1979 (BMDEFS79). Use as the covariate a measure of the women's attitudes toward traditional roles for women in 1979 (BMTRAD79).

 Use the printout from the analysis of covariance to answer the following questions:

a. What was the value of the F statistic for the covariate? Was the value of F statistically significant at the .05 level? What was the exact probability value?
b. What was the value of the F statistic for the main effect? Was the value of F statistically significant at the .05 level? What was the exact probability value?
c. After controlling for BMTRAD79, what were the mean desired family sizes for the three groups of women; i.e., what were the adjusted means?

---

[1] Strictly speaking, BCRACE defines the *Child's* race/ethnicity and not the mother's; the variable is used as a proxy for the mother's race/ethnicity.

SPSS Tip ————————————————————————

In SPSS/PC, analysis of covariance is performed via the ANOVA program, as in the following example:

ANOVA VARIABLES=DV BY IV (1,2) WITH COVAR
  /STATISTICS=1.

This command instructs the computer to perform an ANCOVA in which DV is the dependent variable and IV (a variable whose minimum is 1 and maximum is 2) is the independent variable. Variables specified after WITH (here, only COVAR) are covariates. The STATISTICS=1 subcommand instructs the computer to perform a multiple classification analysis.

———————————————————————————————————————

d. Which racial/ethnic group had the smallest mean desired family size? Can we conclude that this mean is significantly different from the other two means?
e. How much variance in desired family size was accounted for by BMTRAD79 and BCRACE?
f. Assuming a .05 level of significance, state your conclusion based on the ANCOVA, as it might be written for a research report.

   2. The NLSY data set includes a measure of the young mothers' desired family size (BMDEFS79) *and* their ideal family size—the number of children they believe to be ideal for a family (BMIDFS79). Controlling for traditional gender role attitudes (BCTRAD79), test for ethnic/racial differences in BMDEFS79 and BMIDFS79 using MANCOVA. Perform a stepdown analysis in connection with the MANCOVA.
   Use the printout from the MANCOVA to answer the following questions:

a. How many cases are in the MANCOVA analysis?
b. What is the effect of BCRACE and BMTRAD79, taken together, on the composite dependent variable, using Pillai's criterion as the test statistic? Is the criterion statistically significant at conventional levels?
c. Focusing on the results relating to the effect of BCRACE on the two dependent variables (the main MANCOVA results), what is the value of Pillai's criterion? What is the value of Wilks' lambda? Are either of these criteria statistically significant at conventional levels?

SPSS Tip

In SPSS/PC, the MANOVA program is highly complex. Only a few basic instructions are noted here; the SPSS manual can be consulted for information on more complex options. The following is an example of instructions for a simple MANCOVA:

MANOVA DV1 DV2 BY IV (1,3) WITH COVAR
   /PRINT=CELLINFO SIGNIF (STEPDOWN).

The MANOVA command instructs the computer to perform a MANCOVA for the dependent variables DV1 and DV2. The independent variable IV has a minimum value of 1 and a maximum value of 3, shown in parentheses. The covariate (here, named COVAR) is specified after WITH. The PRINT subcommand can be used to produce various statistics. Here, the keyword CELLINFO requests means and *SD*s to be printed for all dependent variables and covariates for every level of the independent variable. The keywords SIGNIF (STEPDOWN) request a stepdown analysis.

---

d. Based on the stepdown analysis, was one dependent variable exclusively responsible for the rejection of the null hypothesis?
e. Assuming a .05 level of significance, state the conclusion based on the MANCOVA, as it might be written for a research report.

   3. Expanding on the multiple regression analysis performed in Chapter 10, perform a canonical analysis with the following two sets of variables:

Dependent variable set (birth outcomes)

PRBWT	Child's birth weight
PRBLENG	Child's length at birth
PRGESTAT	Child's length of gestation in weeks

Independent variable set

NOSMOKE	Whether mother smoked or not during pregnancy
PRWTBEF	Mother's weight before the pregnancy in pounds
PRWTGAIN	Number of pounds mother gained during pregnancy
PRMOCARE	Month in which prenatal care began

SPSS Tip

In SPSS/PC, canonical analysis is performed through the MANOVA program. Due to the complexity of canonical analysis, only the most basic SPSS instructions are noted here; the SPSS manual can be consulted for information on more complex options. The following is an example of instructions for a simple canonical analysis:

```
MANOVA DV1 DV2 WITH IV1 IV2
  /DISCRIM=STAN COR
  /PRINT=SIGNIF (EIGEN DIMENR).
```

Through the DISCRIM subcommand, the MANOVA program will perform a canonical analysis with two sets of variables: variables named to the left of WITH on the one hand (DV1 and DV2) and variables named to the right of WITH on the other hand (IV1 and IV2). The keyword STAN instructs the computer to print standardized canonical weights, and the keyword COR produces structure coefficients. The EIGEN keyword on the PRINT subcommand produces the canonical correlation coefficients, and the keyword DIMENR yields a dimension reduction analysis (the peel-away procedure).

In connection with the canonical analysis, perform a dimension reduction analysis (peel-away procedure) to determine which roots are significant.

Use the printout from the canonical analysis to answer the following questions:

a. What is the value of the Wilks' lambda criterion for testing the null hypothesis that all R_cs as a set are zero in the population? What is the probability value associated with lambda?

b. How many roots were initially extracted? What is the value of all R_cs? According to the dimension reduction analysis, how many roots are statistically significant at $p = .05$ or lower?

c. What are the canonical weights associated with PRBWT on the roots? What are the canonical weights associated with NOSMOKE on the roots?

d. Which variable in the dependent variable set has the highest loading on the first root and what is that loading? Which variable in the dependent variable set has the highest loading on the second root and what is that loading?

e. Which variable in the independent variable set has the highest loading on the first root and what is that loading? Which variable in the independent variable set has the highest loading on the second root and what is that loading?

f. Interpret the pattern of structure coefficients.

B. INDEPENDENT COMPUTER EXERCISES

Use the NLSY data set to perform independent analyses of the type discussed in Chapter 11 of the textbook. Some specific suggestions follow.

1. Rerun one of the analyses performed for Exercise B.1 of Chapter 7 (one-way ANOVAs), *but* run it as an analysis of covariance with at least one interval-level or ratio-level covariate. Select a covariate that you believe is correlated with the dependent variable and that would be useful to control. Do your conclusions about the null hypothesis change as a result of having a covariate? Is the covariate significantly correlated with the dependent variable? Are the adjusted means for the groups substantially different from the unadjusted means? Assuming a .05 level of significance, state your conclusions based on the ANCOVA, as they might be written for a research report.

2. Building upon Exercise B.1 in this chapter, select a variable that is amenable to dummy coding and that could be used as an additional covariate in an ANCOVA. Code the variable and rerun the ANCOVA. Address the questions in Exercise B.1 based on the new analysis. Now, instead of using the dummy variable as a covariate, use it as a second independent variable in a two-way ANCOVA. How, if at all, do the results differ?

3. Building upon either Exercise B.1 or Exercise B.2, select a second dependent variable and run a MANCOVA. What is the effect of the independent variable and covariate, taken together, on the composite dependent variable? Holding the covariate constant, is the independent variable significantly related to the composite dependent variable? If the null hypothesis of no effect is rejected, is one dependent variable exclusively responsible for the rejection of the null hypothesis? Assuming a .05 level of significance, state the conclusion based on the MANCOVA, as it might be written for a research report.

4. Rerun the multiple regression analysis performed for Exercise B.1 or Exercise B.2 of Chapter 10, but add one or more dependent variables to the analysis—in other words, perform a canonical analysis. How many roots are there, and how many are statistically significant? Interpret the dimensionality of the results.

C. EXERCISES IN READING COMPUTER PRINTOUTS

The exercises in this section are based on printouts from a longitudinal study of over 2000 teenage mothers. Use the printouts to answer the questions included in the exercises.

1. Figure 11–1 presents an SPSS/PC printout for an analysis of covariance. The dependent variable is MWARMTH, a maternal warmth/responsiveness scale. The scale is intended to tap the young mother's emotional warmth and nurturance toward her child and her readiness to respond to the child's emotional needs (higher scores reflect greater warmth). The independent variable is DEPRESS, a three-category variable indi-

* * * A N A L Y S I S   O F   V A R I A N C E * * *

MWARMTH   MATERNAL WARMTH SCALE SCORE
BY   DEPRESS   AT RISK OF CLINICL DEPRESSN-FRM CESD SCA
WITH NKIDS   NUMBER OF CHILDREN

Source of Variation	Sum of Squares	DF	Mean Square	F	Signif of F
Covariates	509.870	1	509.870	13.617	.000
NKIDS	509.870	1	509.870	13.617	.000
Main Effects	1034.215	2	517.107	13.811	.000
DEPRESS	1034.215	2	517.107	13.811	.000
Explained	1544.085	3	514.695	13.746	.000
Residual	75633.913	2020	37.443		
Total	77177.998	2023	38.150		

2106 Cases were processed.
   82 Cases (3.9 PCT) were missing.
----

* * * M U L T I P L E   C L A S S I F I C A T I O N   A N A L Y S I S * * *

MWARMTH   MATERNAL WARMTH SCALE SCORE
By   DEPRESS   AT RISK OF CLINICL DEPRESSN-FRM CESD SCA
With NKIDS   NUMBER OF CHILDREN

Grand Mean =   23.501

Variable + Category	N	Unadjusted Dev'n	Eta	Adjusted for Independents Dev'n	Beta	Adjusted for Independents + Covariates Dev'n	Beta
DEPRESS							
0 NOT AT RISK	1213	.55				.54	
1 AT RISK	435	-.41				-.43	
2 AT HIGH RISK	376	-1.30				-1.26	
			.12				.12
Multiple R Squared							.020
Multiple R							.141

FIGURE 11–1. SPSS/PC PRINTOUT FOR EXERCISE C.1

cating the degree to which the young mother is at risk of clinical depression. The covariate is NKIDS, the number of children the young mother has living with her. The ANCOVA tests the null hypothesis that the young mother's warmth as a parent is unrelated to her level of depression:

H_0: $\mu_{\text{MWARMTH for DEPRESS(1)}} = \mu_{\text{MWARMTH for DEPRESS(2)}} = \mu_{\text{MWARMTH for DEPRESS(3)}}$

Use the printout in Figure 11–1 to answer the following questions:

a. What is the value of the F statistic for the covariate? Is the value of F statistically significant at the .05 level? What is the exact probability value?
b. What is the value of the F statistic for the main effect? Can the null hypothesis be rejected at the .05 level of significance? What is the exact probability value?
c. After controlling for NKIDS, what are the mean scores on MWARMTH for the three groups of women; i.e., what are the adjusted means?
d. Which group has the lowest scores on the maternal warmth scale? Can we conclude that this mean is significantly different from the other two means based on the printout?
e. Assuming a .05 level of significance, state your conclusion based on the ANCOVA, as it might be written for a research report.

2. Figure 11–2 shows a portion of an SPSS/PC printout for a MANCOVA (certain panels have been omitted to conserve space). The analysis expands on the analysis described in exercise C.1 in this chapter; a second dependent variable (MCONTROL) has been added to the analysis. The maternal control/responsiveness scale is intended to measure the young mother's authoritarian control over her child, versus a more democratic or permissive style of raising and disciplining a child. Use the printout in Figure 11–2 to answer the following questions:

a. Panel A shows the result of the Box M test for homogeneity of the variance-covariance matrices. What is the value of M? Is M significant at conventional levels? What should the analyst conclude?
b. What is the effect of NKIDS and DEPRESS, taken together, on the composite dependent variable, using Pillai's criterion as the test statistic (panel B)? Is the criterion statistically significant at conventional levels?
c. Focusing on the results relating to the effect of DEPRESS on the two dependent variables (the main MANCOVA results, in panel C), what is the value of Pillai's criterion? What is the value of Wilks' lambda? Are either of these criteria statistically significant at conventional levels?
d. What does the stepdown analysis (panel D) indicate?
e. Assuming a .05 level of significance, state the conclusion based on the MANCOVA, as it might be written for a research report.

A Multivariate test for Homogeneity of Dispersion matrices

    Boxs M =   28.41070
    F WITH (12,5542781) DF =   2.36065, P =   .005 (Approx.)
    Chi-Square with 12 DF =   28.32784, P =   .005 (Approx.)

    - - - - - - - - -

B * * ANALYSIS OF VARIANCE -- DESIGN   1 * *

    EFFECT .. WITHIN CELLS Regression
    Multivariate Tests of Significance (S = 1, M = 0, N = 987)

Test Name	Value	Approx. F	Hypoth. DF	Error DF	Sig. of F
Pillais	.01399	14.01893	2.00	1976.00	.000
Hotellings	.01419	14.01893	2.00	1976.00	.000
Wilks	.98601	14.01893	2.00	1976.00	.000
Roys	.01399				

C * * ANALYSIS OF VARIANCE -- DESIGN   1 * *

    EFFECT .. DEPRESS
    Multivariate Tests of Significance (S = 2, M = -1/2, N = 987)

Test Name	Value	Approx. F	Hypoth. DF	Error DF	Sig. of F
Pillais	.68714	517.37575	4.00	3954.00	.000
Hotellings	2.19505	1083.80700	4.00	3950.00	.000
Wilks	.31295	778.10639	4.00	3952.00	.000
Roys	.68700				

    - - - - - - - - - -
    Univariate F-tests with (2,1977) D. F.

Variable	Hypoth. SS	Error SS	Hypoth. MS	Error MS	F	Sig. of F
MWARMTH	154076.238	74423.1602	77038.1188	37.64449	2046.46458	.000
MCONTROL	66691.8726	280636.219	33345.9363	141.95054	234.91236	.000

    - - - - - - - - - -
D Roy-Bargmann Stepdown F - tests

Variable	Hypoth. MS	Error MS	StepDown F	Hypoth. DF	Error DF	Sig. of F
MWARMTH	77038.1188	37.64449	2046.46458	2	1977	.000
MCONTROL	5665.78591	140.75569	40.25262	2	1976	.000

FIGURE 11–2. SPSS/PC PRINTOUT FOR EXERCISE C.2

3. Figure 11–3 presents a small portion of an SPSS/PC printout for a canonical analysis. The first set of variables (labeled DEPENDENT on the printout) are MWARMTH and MCONTROL, the same two variables used as the dependent variables in the MANCOVA in Exercise C.2. The second set of variables (labeled COVARIATES on the printout) are as follows:

NKIDS	The number of children of the young mother
PARTNR	Whether the mother is living with a husband or partner (0 = no, 1 = yes)
TESTSCOR	Mother's score on a reading test
DIPLOMA	Whether the mother has a high school diploma (0 = no, 1 = yes)
CESD	Mother's full score on the CES-D depression scale

Use Figure 11–3 to answer the following questions:

a. What is the value of Pillai's criterion (panel A) for testing the null hypothesis that all R_cs as a set are zero in the population? What is the probability value associated with this criterion?
b. How many roots are initially extracted (panel B)? What is the value of all R_cs? What proportion of variance is accounted for by the first root?
c. According to the dimension reduction analysis (panel C), how many roots are statistically significant at $p = .05$ or lower? What is the value of Wilks' λ for the first root?
d. Which variable in the dependent variable set (panel D) has the highest loading on the first root and what is that loading? Which variable in the dependent variable set has the highest loading on the second root and what is that loading?
e. Which variable in the second variable set (panel E) has the highest loading on the first root and what is that loading? Which variable in the second variable set has the highest loading on the second root and what is that loading?
f. Interpret the pattern of structure coefficients.

A * * ANALYSIS OF VARIANCE -- DESIGN 1 * *

EFFECT .. WITHIN CELLS Regression
Multivariate Tests of Significance (S = 2, M = 1 , N = 976 1/2)

Test Name	Value	Approx. F	Hypoth. DF	Error DF	Sig. of F
Pillais	.13665	28.68896	10.00	3912.00	.000
Hotellings	.15212	29.72343	10.00	3908.00	.000
Wilks	.86582	29.20613	10.00	3910.00	.000
Roys	.11518				

- - - - - - - - -

B Eigenvalues and Canonical Correlations

Root No.	Eigenvalue	Pct.	Cum. Pct.	Canon Cor.	Sq. Cor
1	.130	85.579	85.579	.339	.115
2	.022	14.421	100.000	.147	.021

- - - - - - - - -

C Dimension Reduction Analysis

Roots	Wilks L.	F	Hypoth. DF	Error DF	Sig. of F
1 TO 2	.86582	29.20613	10.00	3910.00	.000
2 TO 2	.97853	10.72685	4.00	1956.00	.000

D Correlations between DEPENDENT and canonical variables
            Function No.

Variable	1	2
MWARMTH	-.212	.977
MCONTROL	.960	.278

- - - - - - - - -

E Correlations between COVARIATES and canonical variables
            CAN. VAR.

Covariate	1	2
NKIDS	.303	-.416
PARTNR	-.286	-.339
TESTSCOR	-.731	-.227
DIPLOMA	-.650	-.340
CESD	.503	-.684

- - - - - - - - -

FIGURE 11–3. SPSS/PC PRINTOUT FOR EXERCISE C.3

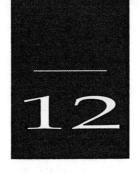

Factor Analysis

A. DIRECTED COMPUTER EXERCISES

Appendixes A, B, and C of this Manual list all the variables in the NLSY data set contained on the enclosed diskette. Perform the analyses described in the following exercises using the NLSY data set, and then answer the accompanying questions. NOTE: Although the NLSY extract data set prepared for this manual includes numerous variables, it is not a data set rich in factor analytic possibilities. Strictly speaking, the factor analyses we propose in this section are not appropriate because all variables are dichotomous. The analyses are included primarily for heuristic purposes.

1. Are there different dimensions to a woman's health-related practices during a pregnancy? To address this question, perform a principal components factor analysis with varimax rotation, using the following variables from the NLSY data set:

PRTRIM1 Had prenatal care first trimester (1 = yes, 0 = no)
NOALC[1] Did not use alcohol during the pregnancy (1) versus *did* use alcohol (0)
NOSMOKE[2] Did not smoke during the pregnancy (1) versus *did* smoke (0)
PRVITAMN Took vitamins during pregnancy (1 = yes, 0 = no)
PRCALOR Reduced calories during the pregnancy (1 = yes, 0 = no)
PRSALT Reduced salt intake during the pregnancy (1 = yes, 0 = no)

Use a minimum eigenvalue of 1.0 as the criterion for number of factors.

---

[1]This dichotomous variable must be created from the original variable PRALCUSE.
[2]This dichotomous variable must be created from the original variable PRSMOKE.

SPSS Tip

In SPSS/PC, factor analyses are performed using the FACTOR procedure. The defaults in SPSS (i.e., the specifications that are automatically in effect unless they are overridden by the analyst) are for a principal components method of extraction; a minimum eigenvalue of 1.0 for number of factors; and the varimax method of factor rotation. Thus, the most basic specification is as follows:

FACTOR VARIABLES=VAR1 TO VAR10.

This command will produce a principal components factor analysis for the 10 named variables.

When you have produced the printout, use it to answer the following questions:

a. How many factors meet the criterion of a minimum eigenvalue of 1.0? What percentage of variance, cumulatively, do these factors account for?
b. Examining the final statistics for the retained factors, what is the variable with the highest communality? What is the variable with the lowest communality?
c. Examining the rotated factor matrix, which variables have high loadings on the first factor and what are those loadings? Which variables have high loadings on subsequent factors and what are those loadings?
d. What should the "names" of the factors be; i.e., what are the underlying dimensions?

2. Is the factor structure achieved in Exercise A.1 stable? Redo the principal components factor analysis as described in Exercise A.1, but do the factor analysis twice, for two random half-samples of the NLSY sample. Then do a factor comparison, using informal procedures, to determine if the factor structure is stable.

When you have produced the printouts, use them to answer the following questions:

a. How many factors were extracted with a minimum eigenvalue of 1.0 for the first random half-sample? For the second random half-sample?
b. What percentage of variance was accounted for by these factors in the first random half-sample? In the second random half-sample?
c. What variables have high loadings on the factors in the first random half-sample? In the second random half-sample? Would the same names be used to label the factors in the two analyses?

SPSS Tip ——————————————————

In SPSS/PC, the SAMPLE command draws a temporary subsample, at random, that is used in the subsequent procedure. The proportion of cases (or the number of cases) must be specified, as in the following example:

SAMPLE .33.
FACTOR VARIABLES=VAR1 TO VAR10.

This command instructs the computer to randomly select one-third of the cases and to use those cases in the specified factor analysis. A second identical SAMPLE command would draw a *different* random subsample of one-third of the cases.

———————————————————————————————

    d. What do you conclude about the stability of the factor structure, based on the overall similarity or dissimilarity of the two solutions?

    3. Although the principal components analysis for Exercise A.1 yielded an interpretable factor solution, the low eigenvalue for the first factor (not much above 1.0) suggests that factor analysis might *not* be appropriate for this set of six variables. Produce a correlation matrix for the variables and use the printout to answer the following questions:

    a. How many of the 15 correlation coefficients in the matrix (i.e., 15 unique pairs) are statistically significant at or beyond the .05 level?

    b. What is the highest bivariate correlation in the matrix? How many correlations are below .30?

    c. What do you conclude about the factorability of the correlation matrix?

    4. To further pursue the issue raised in Exercise A.3, perform a factor analysis of the six variables using the *principal factors* method of extraction. Remember that with this method, the initial estimates of communality are the squared multiple correlation coefficients of a variable with all other variables as the predictors, so that communality information will show the interrelatedness of the variables.

    When you have produced the printout, use it to answer the following questions:

    a. Which variable has the highest initial communality (i.e., the highest R^2 when predicted from all other variables)? What is that communality?

SPSS Tip

Since the principal components method of extraction is the default in SPSS, alternative extraction methods must be specified, as in the following example:

```
FACTOR VARIABLES=VAR1 TO VAR10
  /EXTRACTION=PAF
  /ROTATION=VARIMAX.
```

These instructions will result in a principal factor extraction (PAF) of VAR1 to VAR10 with varimax rotation. (When the EXTRACTION command is used to override the default, the ROTATION command must be used, even when the default rotation method—varimax—is desired.)

---

b. Which variable has the lowest initial communality (i.e., the lowest R^2 when predicted from all other variables)? What is that communality? What do these communality estimates suggest?
c. In the final solution, what percentage of variance was accounted for cumulatively by the rotated factors?
d. Compare the rotated factor structure for this principal factor solution with that for the principal components solution. What are the similarities and differences?
e. Overall, what can be concluded about the factor analysis of the six variables?

B. INDEPENDENT COMPUTER EXERCISES

Use the NLSY data set to perform independent analyses of the type discussed in Chapter 12 of the textbook (or, if possible, use an alternative data set, given the limitations of the NLSY data set for factor analysis). Some specific suggestions follow.

    1. Identify variables in the NLSY (or alternative) data set that might be suitable for a factor analysis and whose underlying dimensionality you are interested in exploring. Begin by having the computer produce a correlation matrix so that you can determine the likely appropriateness of a factor analytic model.

    2. If you have a correlation matrix that appears factorable, proceed with a principal components analysis with varimax rotation, initially using a minimum eigenvalue of

1.0 as the criterion for number of factors. After inspecting the initial output, determine whether the analysis should be rerun using a different number of factors. What appears to be the underlying dimensionality of the variables in your analysis?

3. Rerun your analysis from Exercise B.2 using oblique rotation. To what extent does the factor structure change? What are the correlations between the factors? Which rotation method results in the greatest clarity of structures?

4. Select a nominal-level variable from the data set that you believe might be related to the variables in the factor analysis and determine if the factor structure is similar across the different groups defined by the nominal-level variable. (Examples in the NLSY include a comparison of structures for males versus female Children, women with a cesarean versus those with a vaginal delivery, and so on.)

C. EXERCISES IN READING COMPUTER PRINTOUTS

The exercises in this section are based on printouts from a longitudinal study of over 2000 teenage mothers. Use the printouts to answer the questions included in the exercises.

1. The Center for Epidemiologic Studies-Depression (CES-D) scale is one of the most widely used measures of depression currently available. It consists of 20 statements (e.g., I was bothered by things that usually don't bother me), to which respondents indicate whether, during the past week, the statement was true rarely (< 1 day), some of the time (1-2 days), a moderate amount of time (3-4 days), or most or all the time (5-7 days). Responses to the 20 items (coded 1, 2, 3, or 4) are added together to form a single scale. But are the CES-D items unidimensional? All of the exercises in this section relate to a factor analysis of the items on the CES-D scale.

Figure 12–1 shows the means and *SD*s of the 20 items, plus a portion of the correlation matrix (items 1 through 7 correlated with all items). Use the printout in Figure 12–1 to answer the following questions:

a. The means for most items are between 1.0 and 2.0. What is the mean for item 16? Why do you suppose this item is different? What are the implications for scoring this item on the full CES-D?

b. Which item or items in the correlation matrix (items 1 through 7) have especially high correlations with other items on the scale? Which item has especially low correlation with other items?

c. Overall, does the pattern of correlations suggest a set of items that are factorable?

2. Figure 12–2 shows the initial statistics for principal axis factoring of the 20 CES-D items. Use the printout to answer the following questions:

a. What is the variable with the highest communality and what is that communality? What is the variable with the lowest communality and what is that communality?

- - - - F A C T O R   A N A L Y S I S - - - -

Analysis Number 1 Listwise deletion of cases with missing values

	Mean	Std Dev	Label
CESD1	1.74549	.91272	BOTHERED BY THINGS THAT DONT BOTHER ME
CESD2	1.78063	.95421	DIDN'T FEEL LIKE EATING, POOR APPETITE
CESD3	1.73647	.97735	CANT SHAKE OFF THE BLUES EVEN W FAM HELP
CESD4	3.13913	1.01725	I FELT AS GOOD AS OTHER PEOPLE
CESD5	1.89269	.94045	HAVING TROUBLE W CONCENTRATION
CESD6	1.95632	1.05749	I FELT DEPRESSED
CESD7	2.57787	1.07922	EVERYTHING I DID WAS AN EFFORT
CESD8	2.91595	1.08851	I FELT HOPEFUL ABOUT THE FUTURE
CESD9	1.54321	.86707	MY LIFE HAD BEEN A FAILURE
CESD10	1.54653	.85753	I FELT FEARFUL
CESD11	1.94160	1.05250	MY SLEEP WAS RESTLESS
CESD12	3.17142	.96374	I WAS HAPPY
CESD13	1.78348	.92914	I TALKED LESS THAN USUAL
CESD14	1.91453	1.05358	I FELT LONELY
CESD15	1.46819	.79618	PEOPLE WERE UNFRIENDLY
CESD16	3.21605	.94572	I ENJOYED LIFE
CESD17	1.60304	.93751	I HAD CRYING SPELLS
CESD18	1.79630	.95594	I FELT SAD
CESD19	1.42830	.79058	I FELT THAT PEOPLE DISLIKED ME
CESD20	1.72080	.88852	I COULD NOT GET GOING

Number of Cases =   2106

Correlation Matrix:

	CESD1	CESD2	CESD3	CESD4	CESD5	CESD6	CESD7
CESD1	1.00000						
CESD2	.25605	1.00000					
CESD3	.45040	.31340	1.00000				
CESD4	-.15474	-.09139	-.23260	1.00000			
CESD5	.33399	.20245	.34238	-.10903	1.00000		
CESD6	.44868	.31346	.57720	-.27212	.43762	1.00000	
CESD7	.04039	-.00785	-.00328	.19372	-.01470	.01589	1.00000
CESD8	-.10904	-.05481	-.17623	.32547	-.08167	-.18561	.21404
CESD9	.30204	.23424	.37138	-.25323	.31213	.46576	-.02187
CESD10	.31801	.23310	.37372	-.18197	.31781	.44910	.02970
CESD11	.28025	.29186	.34987	-.16235	.32195	.39850	.00798
CESD12	-.31979	-.26026	-.42863	.38077	-.30729	-.52031	.12350
CESD13	.23860	.23467	.28659	-.14353	.23599	.32253	.04809
CESD14	.33306	.27195	.45469	-.24067	.33882	.54200	-.02631
CESD15	.19347	.17277	.22823	-.07284	.19085	.21614	.01671
CESD16	-.24832	-.17382	-.34081	.37070	-.24099	-.40857	.14758
CESD17	.39486	.26584	.46231	-.21105	.29435	.52589	-.01545
CESD18	.40662	.29107	.54047	-.25565	.34610	.64864	-.01432
CESD19	.28347	.19829	.34781	-.14974	.27398	.35481	-.01517
CESD20	.31360	.26672	.36053	-.16251	.34958	.40868	.00089

FIGURE 12-1. SPSS/PC PRINTOUT FOR EXERCISE C.1

```
Extraction  1  for Analysis  1, Principal Axis Factoring (PAF)

Initial Statistics:

Variable    Communality  *  Factor   Eigenvalue   Pct of Var   Cum Pct
                         *
CESD1          .30288    *    1        6.77761        33.9         33.9
CESD2          .18104    *    2        1.66416         8.3         42.2
CESD3          .44603    *    3        1.08344         5.4         47.6
CESD4          .24585    *    4         .92160         4.6         52.2
CESD5          .27221    *    5         .85586         4.3         56.5
CESD6          .58802    *    6         .81418         4.1         60.6
CESD7          .09161    *    7         .79385         4.0         64.6
CESD8          .17707    *    8         .76880         3.8         68.4
CESD9          .37669    *    9         .69602         3.5         71.9
CESD10         .35094    *   10         .66282         3.3         75.2
CESD11         .26793    *   11         .64956         3.2         78.4
CESD12         .48401    *   12         .63065         3.2         81.6
CESD13         .19555    *   13         .58576         2.9         84.5
CESD14         .45177    *   14         .55422         2.8         87.3
CESD15         .24418    *   15         .51295         2.6         89.9
CESD16         .41095    *   16         .50621         2.5         92.4
CESD17         .46093    *   17         .45241         2.3         94.7
CESD18         .60951    *   18         .40776         2.0         96.7
CESD19         .39454    *   19         .36568         1.8         98.5
CESD20         .32551    *   20         .29648         1.5        100.0

   PAF Extracted   3 factors.   17 Iterations required.
------------------------------------------------------------------------
```

FIGURE 12–2. SPSS/PC PRINTOUT FOR EXERCISE C.2

b. What is the eigenvalue of the first factor? How many factors have an eigenvalue greater than 1.0? How much variance do these factors account for?
c. How many factors should be extracted based on the minimum eigenvalue criterion? How many factors should be extracted based on percentage of variance considerations? How many factors does the scree test suggest?

3. Figure 12–3 shows the rotated factor matrix (varimax rotation) for the three factors that met the minimum eigenvalue of 1.0 criterion. Use the printout to answer the following questions:

a. Of the 20 items in the CES-D scale, how many have loadings on the first factor that are greater than .30? How many items have loadings that are higher on the first factor than on any other factor; i.e., how many items are more clearly associated with factor 1 than with factors 2 or 3? What does the first factor appear to be capturing?
b. How many items have loadings greater than .30 on the second factor? What does the second factor appear to be capturing? Is there an item on this factor that does not seem to "fit"? If yes, which one?

- - - -   F A C T O R   A N A L Y S I S   - - - -

Varimax   Rotation 1, Extraction 1, Analysis 1 - Kaiser Normalization.

Varimax converged in   6 iterations.

Rotated Factor Matrix:

	FACTOR 1	FACTOR 2	FACTOR 3
CESD6	.78096	-.20351	.10155
CESD18	.70596	-.19717	.26986
CESD3	.65956	-.16632	.13534
CESD14	.61646	-.18330	.22409
CESD17	.61114	-.12333	.25175
CESD1	.55391	-.05929	.11817
CESD10	.52059	-.07375	.31470
CESD20	.49619	-.10167	.30300
CESD11	.49485	-.09402	.15507
CESD5	.49263	-.06297	.15560
CESD9	.47707	-.20997	.36381
CESD2	.41014	-.03468	.11267
CESD13	.40046	-.04534	.17100
CESD16	-.39066	.56143	-.08699
CESD4	-.18919	.55810	-.07461
CESD12	-.50214	.52872	-.11233
CESD8	-.09728	.49868	.02606
CESD7	.09508	.36535	-.01873
CESD19	.33190	-.08552	.69800
CESD15	.21747	.02002	.52553

FIGURE 12–3. SPSS/PC PRINTOUT FOR EXERCISE C.3

c. How many items have loadings greater than .30 on the third factor? How many items have loadings that are higher on the third factor than on any other factor; i.e., how many items are more clearly associated with factor 3 than with factors 1 or 2? What does the third factor appear to be capturing?

4. Figure 12–4 shows the factor matrix when only one factor is retained (note than when there is only one factor, there is no factor rotation). Use the printout to answer the following questions:

a. How many of the 20 items have loadings greater than .30 on the single factor? Which item most clearly does not "belong" on this factor?
b. What do the negative signs on some items (e.g., items 12 and 16) mean?
c. If the CES-D scale were being redeveloped, what would you suggest based on the analyses shown in Figures 12–1 to 12–4?

PAF Extracted   1 factors.   4 Iterations required.

Factor Matrix:

	FACTOR 1
CESD18	.78146
CESD6	.77693
CESD14	.68186
CESD3	.67686
CESD17	.66717
CESD12	-.63879
CESD9	.62077
CESD10	.59492
CESD20	.57922
CESD19	.55691
CESD1	.54328
CESD16	-.54124
CESD11	.51949
CESD5	.50709
CESD13	.42768
CESD2	.40997
CESD15	.37206
CESD4	-.36347
CESD8	-.23081
CESD7	-.04372

FIGURE 12–4. SPSS/PC PRINTOUT FOR EXERCISE C.4

Discriminant Analysis and Logistic Regression

A. DIRECTED COMPUTER EXERCISES

Appendixes A, B, and of this Manual list all the variables in the NLSY data set contained on the enclosed diskette. Perform the analyses described in the following exercises using the NLSY data set, and then answer the accompanying questions.

1. Use direct discriminant analysis to explain variation in whether the focal Child's was breastfed (HLBRFED), based on the following predictor variables:

BMAGE1ST	Age of mother when focal Child was born
BMAFQT80	Mother's score on a standardized aptitude test
BCGENDER	Child's gender
BCRACE	Child's race/ethnicity
PRBWT	Child's birth weight

Remember to dummy code both BCGENDER and BCRACE. (So that the analysis will be comparable to ours, permitting a check against answers in Appendix D, use females as the reference group for BCGENDER and use non-Hispanic, non-African Americans as the reference group for BCRACE.) Allow the probability distribution for the breastfeeding and nonbreastfeeding groups to be 50-50; that is, do not establish any prior probabilities.

SPSS Tip —————————————————————

In SPSS/PC, discriminant analysis is performed using the DSCRIMINANT procedure. A basic direct discriminant analysis can be produced using the following commands:

DSCRIMINANT GROUPS=DV (0,1)
  /VARIABLES=IV1 TO IV4
  /STATISTICS=1, 13.

These commands indicate that the dependent (group) variable is DV, which has a minimum value of 0 and a maximum value of 1. The independent variables are IV1, IV2, IV3, and IV4. The STATISTICS subcommand instructs the computer to produce first, the group means for all independent variables (code 1) and second, a classification table for all cases (code 13).

When you have produced the printout, use it to answer the following questions:

a. How many cases were used in the discriminant analysis? How many of the mothers breastfed the focal Child? Calculate the percentage of women who breastfed.
b. What is the mean birth weight of Children who were breastfed? What is the mean birth weight of Children who were *not* breastfed? What percentage of male Children were breastfed? What percentage of female Children were breastfed?
c. What is the value of Wilks' lambda for the overall discriminant function? What is the probability level associated with this lambda? What percentage of variance in the breastfed/nonbreastfed variable is accounted for by the set of independent variables?
d. Which independent variable has the highest loading on the discriminant function and what is that loading? Which independent variable has the lowest loading on the discriminant function and what is that loading?
e. What are the centroids for the two groups?
f. How many women who *actually* breastfed their infants were predicted to be in the breastfeeding group? What percentage of all breastfeeders were correctly classified? Overall, what percentage of cases were correctly classified based on predicted group membership?

2. Perform another discriminant analysis using the same variables as Exercise A.1. This time, however, crossvalidate the classification by randomly dividing the sample

into two groups. One method of dividing the sample roughly in half in a "random" fashion is to use the variable BMBIRTMO (the month in which the mother was born) to form two subgroups. That is, create a selection variable (SUBGRP) that is equal to 0 for women born in the first 6 months (January to June, codes 1 to 6) and to 1 for those born in the second 6 months (July to December, codes 7 to 12). Also, establish prior probabilities in this discriminant analysis that are proportionate to the distribution of breastfeeding women in the NLSY sample.

When you have produced the printout, use it to answer the following questions:

a. How many cases were used in the discriminant analysis? How many women in this analysis subsample breastfed their infants? Calculate the percentage of women in the analysis subsample who breastfed. What are the prior probabilities for the breastfeeding and nonbreastfeeding groups?

SPSS Tip ────────────────────────────

In SPSS/PC, the DSCRIMINANT program allows for the establishment of prior probabilities and also for the selection of a crossvalidation subsample, as in the following example:

```
DSCRIMINANT GROUPS=DV (0,1)
  /VARIABLES=IV1 TO IV4
  /SELECT=SUBGRP (1)
  /PRIORS=SIZE
  /STATISTICS=1, 13.
```

These commands are comparable to those used in the previous example, except that two subcommands have been added. The SELECT subcommand instructs the computer to develop the discriminant function based only on those cases that have a code of 1 for a previously defined variable named SUBGRP; the cases coded with a value other than 1 will not be used in the basic analysis, but will be used in the classification stage for crossvalidation purposes. The subcommand PRIORS=SIZE sets the probabilities for group membership equal to the proportion of the cases that fall into each group in the analysis.

b. What is the value of Wilks' lambda for the discriminant function for the analysis subsample? What is the probability level associated with this lambda? What percentage of variance in the breastfed/nonbreastfed variable is accounted for by the set of independent variables? Compare these results to those obtained in Exercise A.1.c.

c. Overall, what percentage of cases in the analysis subsample were correctly classified based on predicted group membership? Compare this result to that obtained in Exercise A.1.f.

d. How many cases were in the "unselected" subsample used for purposes of crossvalidation? Overall, what percentage of cases in the crossvalidation subsample were correctly classified? What can be concluded based on the classification results for the two subsamples?

   3. Perform a direct logistic regression to predict the probability of a woman breastfeeding, based on the same predictors used in Exercises A.1 and A.2. Use the same pro-

SPSS Tip ─────────────────────────────────

In SPSS/PC, the LOGISTIC REGRESSION program is used to perform a logistic regression analysis. As with other multivariate procedures, the SPSS program for logistic regression is complex and offers numerous options that are beyond the scope of this book to explain. A basic specification is as follows:

```
LOGISTIC REGRESSION VARIABLES=DV WITH IV1, IV2, IV3
   /SELECT SUBGRP EQ 1.
```

This command instructs the computer to perform a logit analysis that regresses the dependent variable (DV) simultaneously on the three independent variables that follow WITH (IV1, IV2, and IV3). Note that in the LOGISTIC REGRESSION program, the TO convention *cannot* be used to identify the predictor variables (i.e., we could not have specified VARIABLES=DV WITH IV1 TO IV3). The SELECT subcommand instructs the computer to develop the logistic regression equation using only cases for which the variable SUBGRP is coded 1; the cases not coded 1 are used in the classification stage for crossvalidation.

cedure as in Exercise A.2 to split the NLSY sample into two roughly equal subsamples so that the logistic regression classification can be crossvalidated.

When you have produced the printout, use it to answer the following questions:

a. What is the number of selected and unselected cases (prior to rejection due to missing data)? How many cases were used in the analysis?
b. What is the value of $-2 LL$ in the initial function (i.e., with just the constant in the model)? What is the value of $-2 LL$ after the independent variables are entered into the model?
c. What is the value of the model chi-square for the logistic regression analysis? What is the probability value associated with this chi-square?
d. Overall, what percentage of cases were correctly classified based on predicted probabilities for breastfeeding? Was this better, worse, or about the same as with discriminant analysis? What percentage of cases were correctly classified using the crossvalidation sample?
e. Which independent variables were statistically significant predictors of breastfeeding probability? (State both the variables and the *direction* associated with the variables—e.g., were older mothers significantly *less* likely or *more* likely to breastfeed than younger ones?)
f. What is the "relative risk" of being breastfed for male versus female infants; i.e., what is the odds ratio for gender?

B. INDEPENDENT COMPUTER EXERCISES

Use the NLSY data set to perform independent analyses of the type described in Chapter 13 of the textbook. Some specific suggestions follow.

1. Develop a hypothesis for a four-variable discriminant analysis. That is, select a categorical variable—a dichotomous variable is preferable—in the NLSY data set that you would like to predict or explain (Y) and then select three variables (X_1, X_2, and X_3) that you hypothesize would be good predictors. Use direct discriminant analysis to enter the predictor variables. Evaluate the model in terms of statistical significance and accuracy of the resulting classification.

2. Using a hierarchical approach, add one more variable that you believe would significantly improve the predictive ability of the equation specified in Exercise B.1. What is the loading for the new variable? Is the improvement to lambda significant? Compare the percentage of cases correctly classified for the two analyses.

3. Use logistic regression to predict the same dependent variable from Exercise B.2, using the same set of predictors. (Note that if the dependent variable selected for Exercise B.2 is not dichotomous, an alternative model will have to be developed.) Are all variables significant predictors of Y? Is classification better, worse, or the same with logistic regression compared to discriminant analysis?

C. EXERCISES IN READING COMPUTER PRINTOUTS

The exercises in this section are based on printouts from a longitudinal study of over 2000 teenage mothers. Use the printouts to answer the questions included in the exercises.

1. Figure 13–1 presents a printout for a direct discriminant analysis involving the prediction of membership in one of two groups for the variable DRUGUSE, coded 1 if

```
- - - - - - - -   D I S C R I M I N A N T   A N A L Y S I S   - - - - - - - -
```

A On groups defined by DRUGUSE   USE OF ANY DRUG PAST MONTH

```
        2106 (unweighted) cases were processed.
           0 of these were excluded from the analysis.
        2106 (unweighted) cases will be used in the analysis.
```

Number of Cases by Group

DRUGUSE	Number of Cases Unweighted	Weighted	Label
0	1819	1819.0	
1	287	287.0	
Total	2106	2106.0	

Group means

DRUGUSE	ALCOHOL	CESD	DLC
0	.31336	15.40462	2.56185
1	.76655	19.72125	3.57143
Total	.37512	15.99288	2.69943

B On groups defined by DRUGUSE   USE OF ANY DRUG PAST MONTH

```
Analysis number         1
Direct method:  All variables passing the tolerance test are entered.
        Minimum Tolerance Level.................. .00100
```

Canonical Discriminant Functions

```
        Maximum number of functions.............       1
        Minimum cumulative percent of variance... 100.00
        Maximum significance of Wilks' Lambda.... 1.0000
```

Prior Probabilities

Group	Prior	Label
0	.86372	
1	.13628	
Total	1.00000	

Canonical Discriminant Functions

C

Fcn	Eigenvalue	Pct of Variance	Cum Pct	Canonical Corr	:	After Fcn	Wilks' Lambda	Chisquare	DF	Sig
					:	0	.8718	288.429	3	.0000
1*	.1470	100.00	100.00	.3580	:					

* marks the   1 canonical discriminant functions remaining in the analysis.

FIGURE 13–1. SPSS/PC PRINTOUT FOR EXERCISE C.1

D Standardized Canonical Discriminant Function Coefficients

```
            FUNC  1
ALCOHOL     .84430
CESD        .19049
DLC         .35631
```

Structure Matrix:

Pooled-within-groups correlations between discriminating variables
                                and canonical discriminant functions
E (Variables ordered by size of correlation within function)

```
            FUNC  1
ALCOHOL     .88434
DLC         .51219
CESD        .37194
```

Unstandardized Canonical Discriminant Function Coefficients

```
            FUNC  1
ALCOHOL     1.840540
CESD        .1833649E-01
DLC         .2019446
(constant)  -1.528810
```

Canonical Discriminant Functions evaluated at Group Means (Group Centroids)

```
Group       FUNC  1
  0         -.15224
  1          .96491
```

F Classification Results -

Actual Group	No. of Cases	Predicted Group Membership 0	1
Group 0	1819	1798 98.8%	21 1.2%
Group 1	287	262 91.3%	25 8.7%

Percent of "grouped" cases correctly classified: 86.56%

FIGURE 13–1 (CONT.)

the woman used drugs (marijuana, cocaine, crack, heroin, PCP, etc.) at least once in the previous 30 days, and coded 0 if she did not use drugs. The three predictor variables in the analysis are:

ALCOHOL Woman got high on alcohol at least once in previous 30 days (1 = yes, 0 = no)

CESD Score on CES-D depression scale (higher scores = higher level of depression)

DLC Score on Difficult Life Circumstances scale (higher scores = higher daily stresses/problems)

Use the printout to answer the following questions:

a. How many cases were used in the discriminant analysis? How many of the women had used any type of drug in the month prior to the interview (panel A)?

b. What is the mean depression score for women who used drugs? What is the mean depression score for women who did *not* use drugs? What percentage of women who used drugs had gotten high on alcohol in the previous month? What percentage of women who did *not* use drugs had gotten high on alcohol in the previous month?

c. Were prior probabilities used in the analysis? At what values were the probabilities set (panel B)?

d. What is the value of Wilks' lambda for the overall discriminant function and what is the probability level associated with this lambda? What is the canonical correlation coefficient? Compute the percentage of variance in drug use status accounted for by the predictors, using both the canonical correlation and lambda (panel C).

e. What is the equation for the unstandardized discriminant function (panel D)?

f. With which independent variable are discriminant function scores most highly correlated? What is the loading for that variable? Which independent variables have loadings that are greater than .30 (Panel E)?

g. How many women were falsely predicted to have used drugs? What percentage of women who actually used drugs were correctly classified? Overall, what percentage of all cases were correctly classified based on predicted group membership (Panel F)?

2. Figure 13–2 presents a portion of a printout for a stepwise discriminant analysis that is similar in many respects to the analysis for Exercise C.1. That is, the dependent variable is DRUGUSE and three of the predictor variables are ALCOHOL, DLC, and CESD. In addition, two other independent variables have been included:

NSUPPORT   Number of people the woman has available to her as social supports

MASTERY   Score on a scale measuring mastery/self-efficacy (higher scores = greater perceived self-efficacy)

Figure 13–2 shows the printout at the fourth step of the analysis—i.e., after three variables have already entered the discriminant equation. Use the printout to answer the following questions:

a. Which variable was entered on the fourth step? What was the value of lambda at that point? What was the F value associated with lambda? At that point, what was the overall level of significance for the discriminant function (panel A)?

b. Which variables were already in the equation at step 4; i.e., what variables were entered on the first three steps? Which variable was stepped in first? What was the value of lambda after the first variable was entered?

c. Which variable was *not* in the equation at step 4? What was the value of the F to enter this last variable? Did this variable enter the equation in a subsequent step?

d. What was the canonical correlation for the final analysis? What percentage of variance in drug use status was accounted for by the predictors (panel B)?

e. Is having more social supports associated with an increased likelihood or a decreased likelihood of drug use (panel C)?

f. In this analysis, how many women were falsely predicted to have used drugs? Overall, what percentage of cases were correctly classified based on predicted group membership? Compare this to the percentage of correctly classified cases in Exercise C.1 (panel D).

A At step   4, NSUPPORT was included in the analysis.

		Degrees of Freedom	Signif.	Between Groups
Wilks' Lambda	.87167	4 1 2096.0		
Equivalent F	77.0358	4 2093.0	.0000	

----------------- Variables in the analysis after step   4 -----------------

Variable	Tolerance	F to remove	Wilks' Lambda
ALCOHOL	.9914783	206.11	.95751
CESD	.8025275	7.2190	.87467
DLC	.8213420	28.916	.88371
NSUPPORT	.9676903	1.3807	.87224

----------------- Variables not in the analysis after step   4 -----------------

Variable	Tolerance	Minimum Tolerance	F to enter	Wilks' Lambda
MASTERY	.7529458	.6543096	.56828	.87143

F statistics and significances between pairs of groups after step   4
Each F statistic has   4 and   2093.0 degrees of freedom.

                    Group   0

    Group
        1   77.036
                           .0000

F level or tolerance or VIN insufficient for further computation.

                            Summary Table

	Action		Vars	Wilks'		
Step	Entered	Removed	In	Lambda	Sig.	Label
1	ALCOHOL		1	.89786	.0000	GOT HIGH ON ALCOHOL PAST MONTH
2	DLC		2	.87585	.0000	DIFFICULT LIFE CIRCS SCALE
3	CESD		3	.87224	.0000	CESD DEPRESSION SCALE
4	NSUPPORT		4	.87167	.0000	AVAILABLE SOCIAL SUPPORTS

B   Canonical Discriminant Functions

		Pct of	Cum	Canonical	After	Wilks'			
Fcn	Eigenvalue	Variance	Pct	Corr	Fcn	Lambda	Chisquare	DF	Sig
					: 0	.8717	287.603	4	.0000
1*	.1472	100.00	100.00	.3582 :					

   * marks the   1 canonical discriminant functions remaining in the analysis.

FIGURE 13–2. SPSS/PC PRINTOUT FOR EXERCISE C.2

Continued

C Standardized Canonical Discriminant Function Coefficients

```
              FUNC  1
ALCOHOL       .83939
CESD          .18269
DLC           .35957
NSUPPORT     -.07286
```

Structure Matrix:

Pooled-within-groups correlations between discriminating variables
                              and canonical discriminant functions
(Variables ordered by size of correlation within function)

```
              FUNC  1
ALCOHOL       .87901
DLC           .51440
CESD          .37911
MASTERY      -.21060
NSUPPORT     -.10919
```

Canonical Discriminant Functions evaluated at Group Means (Group Centroids)

```
    Group     FUNC  1
      0       -.15237
      1        .96534
```

D Classification Results –

Actual Group	No. of Cases	Predicted Group Membership 0	1
Group 0	1812	1793 99.0%	19 1.0%
Group 1	286	262 91.6%	24 8.4%

Percent of "grouped" cases correctly classified: 86.61%

FIGURE 13–2 (CONT.)

3. Figure 13–3 presents a portion of a printout[1] for a logistic regression analysis in which the dependent variable is the same as that used in the previous exercises (DRUGUSE). The independent variables are ALCOHOL and CESD, as well as PROB1 to PROB10, which are dichotomous variables indicating whether or not the mother was experiencing specific stresses—the items that form the Difficult Life Circumstances scale. The 10 stresses (all coded 1 if yes, 0 if no) are as follows:

PROB1   Do you have arguments most days with your present boyfriend/husband?
PROB2   Are you having some sort of problem with any former boyfriends or a former husband?

---

[1] Omitted from the printout is the information on number of cases used in the analysis (2106), the listing of the independent variables, and the value of –2 *LL* prior to entering independent variables (1676.9982).

PROB3   Do you have a relative or boyfriend who is in jail?

PROB4   Do you get hassled pretty often by bill collectors or collection agencies?

PROB5   Do you have people living with you who you wish weren't there or who you wish you didn't have to live with?

PROB6   Do you have neighbors who are giving you or your children any kind of problem?

PROB7   Does someone you are close to have a problem with alcohol or drugs?

PROB8   Has someone you were close to died or been killed in the last year?

PROB9   Have you been robbed, mugged, or attacked in the past year?

PROB10   Have you had trouble in the past year finding a good place to live?

Use the printout to answer the following questions:

a. What is the value of $-2 LL$ after the independent variables are entered into the model? What is the value of the chi-square statistic, and what is the probability level associated with this chi-square (panel A)?

A   SPSS/PC PRINTOUT FOR EXERCISE C.3

```
Dependent Variable..   DRUGUSE    USE OF ANY DRUG PAST MONTH

Beginning Block Number  0.   Initial Log Likelihood Function

-2 Log Likelihood    1676.9982

* Constant is included in the model.


Beginning Block Number  1.  Method: Enter

Variable(s) Entered on Step Number
1..       ALCOHOL    GOT HIGH ON ALCOHOL PAST MONTH
          CESD       CESD DEPRESSION SCALE
          PROB1      ARGUMENTS MOST DAYS W PARTNER
          PROB2      ARGUMENTS W FORMER PARTNER
          PROB3      SOMEONE CLOSE IN JAIL
          PROB4      HASSLED BY BILL COLLECTORS
          PROB5      RATHER NOT LIVE W HOUSEHOLD MEMBERS
          PROB6      AGGRAVATING NEIGHBORS
          PROB7      SOMEONE CLOSE HAS DRUG-ALC PROB
          PROB8      SOMEONE CLOSE DIED PAST YR
          PROB9      BEEN ROBBED OR MUGGED PAST YR
          PROB10     TROUBLE FINDING GOOD PLACE TO LIVE

Estimation terminated at iteration number 5 because
Log Likelihood decreased by less than .01 percent.

    -2 Log Likelihood      1399.157
    Goodness of Fit        2035.182
                           Chi-Square    df Significance
    Model Chi-Square        277.841      12      .0000
    Improvement             277.841      12      .0000
```

FIGURE 13–3. SPSS/PC PRINTOUT FOR EXERCISE C.3

Continued

B Classification Table for DRUGUSE

```
                    Predicted
              .00      1.00     Percent Correct
               0    |    1
 Observed         +--------+--------+
   .00       0    |  1800  |   19   |    98.96%
                  +--------+--------+
  1.00       1    |   270  |   17   |     5.92%
                  +--------+--------+
                        Overall   86.28%
```

C --------------------- Variables in the Equation ---------------------

Variable	B	S.E.	Wald	df	Sig	R	Exp(B)
ALCOHOL	1..9035	.1521	156.7159	1	.0000	.3037	6.7094
CESD	.0196	.0070	7.7240	1	.0054	.0584	1.0198
PROB1	.3356	.1425	5.5432	1	.0186	.0460	1.3987
PROB2	.1071	.1498	.5108	1	.4748	.0000	1.1130
PROB3	.3477	.1513	5.2840	1	.0215	.0443	1.4158
PROB4	.0117	.1499	.0061	1	.9380	.0000	1.0117
PROB5	.0196	.1742	.0126	1	.9105	.0000	1.0198
PROB6	.2553	.1991	1.6437	1	.1998	.0000	1.2908
PROB7	.5238	.1499	12.2156	1	.0005	.0780	1.6884
PROB8	.1232	.1421	.7522	1	.3858	.0000	1.1312
PROB9	-.0177	.1903	.0087	1	.9257	.0000	.9824
PROB10	.2138	.1440	2.2069	1	.1374	.0111	1.2384
Constant	-3.8708	.1953	392.9604	1	.0000		

FIGURE 13–3 (CONT.)

b. How many women were falsely predicted to have a high probability of using drugs, based on the logistic regression? What percentage of all women who actually used drugs were correctly classified? Overall, what percentage of cases were correctly classified based on predicted group membership (panel B)?

c. What is the logistic regression equation, rounding coefficients to two decimal places (panel C)?

d. Which independent variables were statistically significant predictors of drug use probability? (State both the variables and the *direction* associated with the variables—e.g., were less depressed women more or less likely to be drug users?)

f. What is the "relative risk" of being a drug user if someone close has a drug/alcohol problem, compared to those who do not have someone close with such a problem; i.e., what is the odds ratio?

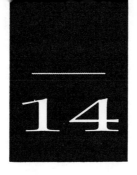

Causal Modeling: Path Analysis and Linear Structural Relations Analysis

A. DIRECTED COMPUTER EXERCISES

Appendixes A, B, and C of this Manual list all the variables in the NLSY data set contained on the enclosed diskette. Perform the analyses described in the following exercises using the NLSY data set, and then answer the accompanying questions.

1. Figure 14–1 presents a hypothesized causal model for explaining the mother's age when she first gave birth (BMAGE1ST) based on three predictor variables:

BMAGEMEN   Mother's age at menarche
BMAFQT80   Score on a standardized aptitude test (cognitive skills)
BMAGEINT   Mother's age at first sexual intercourse

The model postulates that the mothers' age at physiological maturity and their cognitive skills independently affect their age at first intercourse. Age at first intercourse, in turn, is hypothesized to affect the women's age at first birth. Age at menarche and cognitive skills are hypothesized to have both direct effects and indirect effects (through age at first intercourse) on age at first birth. Answer the following questions on the basis of this model:

a. Is the proposed model recursive or nonrecursive?
b. Which variables in the model are endogenous? Which variables are exogenous?

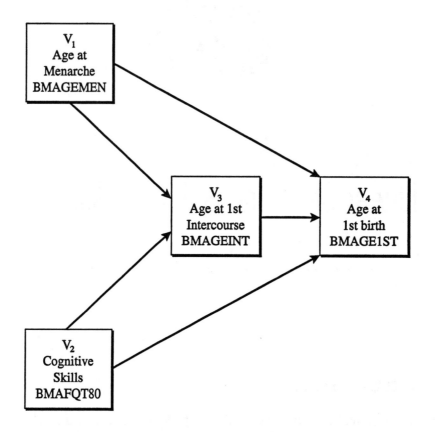

FIGURE 14-1. HYPOTHESIZED CAUSAL MODEL FOR PREDICTING MOTHERS'AGE AT FIRST BIRTH

c. Is the model just-identified, overidentified, or underidentified?
d. Write out the structural equations for this model.
e. How many separate multiple regression analyses would need to be performed to test the proposed model?

2. Using a series of multiple regression analyses, test the causal model that is diagrammed in Figure 14–1.

Use the computer printouts from the regression analyses to answer the following questions:

a. On the path diagram in Figure 14–1, write the correlation coefficients for all the drawn paths.
b. What are the values of R and R^2 for the prediction of BMAGEINT? What is the significance level of this regression?

SPSS Tip

In SPSS/PC, the REGRESSION program allows multiple analyses in a single regression run, as in the following example:

```
REGRESSION VARIABLES=DV IV1 TO IV4
  /STATISTICS=DEFAULTS
  /DESCRIPTIVES=DEFAULTS
  /DEPENDENT=IV4
  /METHOD=ENTER IV1 TO IV3
  /DEPENDENT=DV
  /METHOD=ENTER IV1 TO IV4
```

These commands specify a five-variable analysis with two separate simultaneous multiple regressions (i.e., two separate METHOD subcommands). The first analysis regresses IV4, a mediating variable, on IV1 through IV3. The second regresses the ultimate dependent variable, DV, on the four predictor variables.

---

c. What are the values of R and R^2 for the prediction of BMAGE1ST? What is the significance level of this regression?

d. What are the values of all path coefficients? In a different color pen than used for part a of this exercise, write all the path coefficients on the path diagram in Figure 14–1.

e. Are all paths statistically significant at $p < .05$? What paths, if any, could be trimmed on the basis of a statistical criterion?

f. Calculate the value of e_3 and e_4 in the model.

3. Using a statistical criterion ($p < .05$), trim the causal model based on the results from Exercise A.2 and rerun the regression analyses. Use the printout to answer the following questions:

a. What is the new value of R and R^2 for the prediction of BMAGE1ST? What is the significance level of this regression? How much did R^2 change as a result of theory trimming; i.e., what is the difference for R^2 here and in Exercise A.2?

b. Draw a new path diagram for the trimmed model and write all the path coefficients on the diagram.

c. Are all paths statistically significant? What paths, if any, could be trimmed on the basis of a statistical criterion?

B. INDEPENDENT COMPUTER EXERCISES

Use the NLSY data set to perform independent analyses of the type described in Chapter 14 of the textbook. Some specific suggestions follow.

1. Develop a hypothesized causal model for a three- or four-variable path analysis using the NLSY data. Draw a path diagram and write a one-paragraph statement articulating the proposed causal chain. Respond to the questions in Exercise A.1 with respect to this model.

2. Test the hypothesized model from Exercise B.1 using a series of multiple regression analyses. Examine the results and, if warranted, trim the model and rerun the analyses.

3. Use the results from the final model in Exercise B.2 to attempt to reproduce the correlations in the model. That is, determine the direct and indirect effects of the variables in the analysis. Evaluate the hypothesized causal model on the basis of all the obtained results.

C. EXERCISES IN READING COMPUTER PRINTOUTS

The exercises in this section are based on printouts from a longitudinal study of over 2000 teenage mothers. Use the printouts to answer the questions included in the exercises.

1. Figure 14–2 presents a hypothesized causal model for explaining scores on HOME@TOT—the Home Observation for Measurement of the Environment (HOME) scale, which measures the quality of the focal Child's home environment, based on three predictor variables:

NKIDS   The number of children of the young mother
CESD   Mother's score on the CES-D depression scale
PSTRESS Mother's score on a parenting stress scale

The model postulates that the HOME scores are affected directly by all three predictor variables, and indirectly by NKIDS and CESD through PSTRESS. Answer the following questions on the basis of this model:

a. Which variables in the model are endogenous? Which variables are exogenous?

b. Is the model just-identified, overidentified, or underidentified?

c. Which predictor variables are negatively correlated with HOME scores? Which are positively correlated with HOME scores?

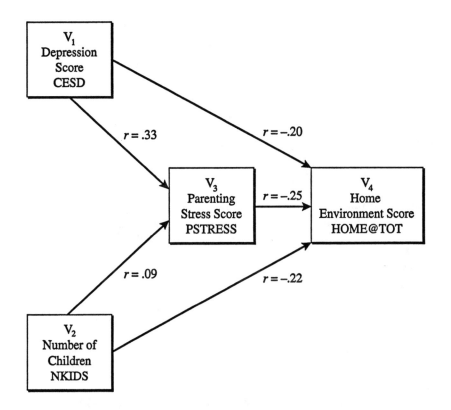

FIGURE 14–2. HYPOTHESIZED CAUSAL MODEL FOR PREDICTING HOME ENVIRONMENT SCORES

d. Describe in words what the correlation between CESD and PSTRESS indicates.
e. How many separate multiple regression analyses would need to be performed to test the proposed model? State what the predictor and dependent variables would be for all regressions.

2. Figure 14–3 presents a portion of a printout for two multiple regression analyses used to test the causal model diagrammed in Figure 14–2. Use the computer printout to answer the following questions:

a. What are the values of R and R^2 for the prediction of PSTRESS? What is the significance level of this regression (panel A)?
b. Are NKIDS and CESD significantly related to PSTRESS at or beyond the .05 level? What is the t value for NKIDS? For CESD?

* * * * M U L T I P L E   R E G R E S S I O N * * * *

A Equation Number 1   Dependent Variable..   PSTRESS   SCORE ON PARENTING STRESS

Block Number 1. Method: Enter   CESD   NKIDS

Variable(s) Entered on Step Number
   1..   NKIDS   NUMBER OF CHILDREN
   2..   CESD   DEPRESSION SCORE 1ST FOLLOWUP

Multiple R   .33943
R Square   .11521
Adjusted R Square   .11427
Standard Error   12.85559

Analysis of Variance

	DF	Sum of Squares	Mean Square
Regression	2	40370.94698	20185.47349
Residual	1876	310039.59054	165.26631

F =   122.13907   Signif F = .0000

------------------ Variables in the Equation ------------------

Variable	B	SE B	Beta	T	Sig T
NKIDS	1.357244	.360551	.081809	3.764	.0002
CESD	.434803	.028952	.326376	15.018	.0000
(Constant)	18.587212	.807321		23.023	.0000

FIGURE 14–3. SPSS/PC PRINTOUT FOR EXERCISE C.2

c. What are the values of R and R^2 for the prediction of HOME@TOT? What is the significance level of this regression (panel B)?
d. What are the values of all path coefficients? Write all the path coefficients on the path diagram in Figure 14–2.
e. Are all paths statistically significant? What paths, if any, could be trimmed on the basis of a statistical criterion?
f. Calculate the value of e_3 and e_4 in the model.
g. How good a job does the causal model do in explaining HOME scores?

3. Figure 14–4 presents a causal model similar to the one proposed in Figure 14–2, except that an additional path has been added—the path between total household earnings (EARNHH) and HOME scale scores. As the figure indicates, there is a modest, positive correlation between household earnings and the measure of the quality of the home environment. Figure 14–5 presents a portion of the regression analysis used to test the revised causal model. Use the computer printout to answer the following questions:

```
* * * *   M U L T I P L E   R E G R E S S I O N   * * * *
```

B Equation Number 2   Dependent Variable..   HOME@TOT   HOME ENVIRONMT SCALE TOT

Block Number 1. Method: Enter   CESD   NKIDS   PSTRESS

```
Variable(s) Entered on Step Number
   1..   PSTRESS   SCORE ON PARENTING STRESS SCALE
   2..   NKIDS     NUMBER OF CHILDREN
   3..   CESD      DEPRESSION SCORE 1ST FOLLOWUP
```

```
Multiple R          .33847
R Square            .11456
Adjusted R Square   .11315
Standard Error    14.08844
```

Analysis of Variance

	DF	Sum of Squares	Mean Square
Regression	3	48151.49241	16050.49747
Residual	1875	372157.69901	198.48411

F =   80.86540   Signif F = .0000

------------------ Variables in the Equation ------------------

Variable	B	SE B	Beta	T	Sig T
PSTRESS	-.210379	.025302	-.192091	-8.315	.0000
NKIDS	-3.490426	.396617	-.192098	-8.800	.0000
CESD	-.184546	.033582	-.126484	-5.495	.0000
(Constant)	115.140877	1.001971		114.914	.0000

End Block Number   1   All requested variables entered.

FIGURE 14–3 (CONT.)

a. Would the path coefficients for paths p_{31} and p_{32} change as a result of the alterations to the model, relative to what they were in the previous model?

b. What are the values of R and R^2 for the prediction of HOME@TOT? How much of an improvement to R^2 does the inclusion of EARNHH make over the value of R^2 without this variable?

c. What are the values of all path coefficients? Write all the path coefficients on the path diagram in Figure 14–4.

d. Comment on how good a job the causal model does in explaining HOME scores—both in the absolute and relative to what was achieved without EARNHH?

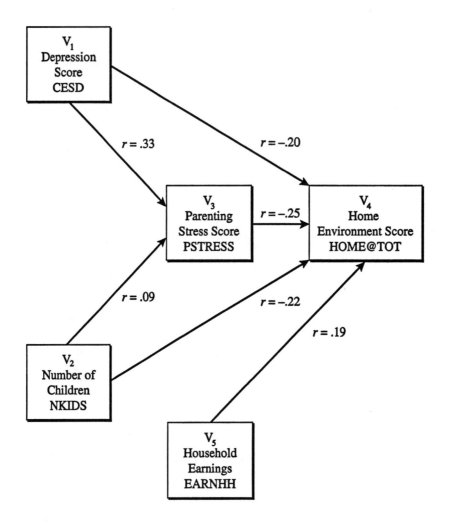

FIGURE 14–4. REVISED HYPOTHESIZED CAUSAL MODEL FOR PREDICTING HOME ENVIRONMENT SCORES

* * * *   M U L T I P L E   R E G R E S S I O N   * * * *

Equation Number 2   Dependent Variable..   HOME@TOT   HOME ENVIRONMT SCALE TOT

Block Number 1. Method: Enter   CESD   NKIDS   PSTRESS   EARNHH

Variable(s) Entered on Step Number
    1..   EARNHH   HOUSEHOLD EARNINGS
    2..   NKIDS   NUMBER OF CHILDREN
    3..   CESD   DEPRESSION SCORE 1ST FOLLOWUP
    4..   PSTRESS   SCORE ON PARENTING STRESS SCALE

Multiple R   .37331
R Square   .13936
Adjusted R Square   .13752
Standard Error   13.89346

Analysis of Variance
                    DF   Sum of Squares   Mean Square
Regression   4   58574.11864   14643.52966
Residual   1874   361735.07277   193.02832

F =   75.86208   Signif F =   .0000

------------------ Variables in the Equation ------------------

Variable	B	SE B	Beta	T	Sig T
EARNHH	.004079	5.55136E-04	.158293	7.348	.0000
NKIDS	-3.373082	.391454	-.185640	-8.617	.0000
CESD	-.172867	.033155	-.118479	-5.214	.0000
PSTRESS	-.200075	.024991	-.182683	-8.006	.0000
(Constant)	113.389725	1.016436		111.556	.0000

FIGURE 14–5. SPSS/PC PRINTOUT FOR EXERCISE C.3

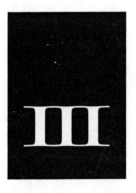

APPENDIXES

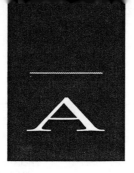

Variables in the NLSY Data File, in Order of Appearance in File

ADMINISTRATIVE VARIABLES (AD)

Variable	Record	Columns	Format	Variable Label
ADID	1	1-4	F4	CASE ID NUMBER
ADINTMO	1	6-7	F2	MONTH OF 1986 INTERVIEW
ADINTYR	1	9-10	F2	YEAR OF 1986 INTERVIEW

BACKGROUND CHARACTERISTICS OF THE CHILD (BC)

Variable	Record	Columns	Format	Variable Label
BCRACE	1	12-13	F2	RACE-ETHNICITY OF CHILD
BCGENDER	1	15-16	F2	GENDER OF CHILD
BCBIRTMO	1	18-19	F2	BIRTH MONTH OF CHILD
BCBIRTYR	1	21-22	F2	BIRTH YEAR OF CHILD
BCAGEMON	1	24-25	F2	CHILD'S AGE IN MONTHS
BCAGE	1	27-28	F2	CHILD'S AGE IN YRS, TRUNCATED
BCGRADE	1	30-31	F2	CHILD'S GRADE IN SCHOOL
BCSPACNG	1	33-34	F2	# MONTHS TO NXT YOUNGER SIBLING OF CHILD
BCHHSIZE	1	36-37	F2	# OF HOUSEHOLD MEMBERS
BCNSIBS	1	39-40	F2	# OF CHILD'S SIBLINGS IN SAME HOUSEHOLD

Variable	Record	Columns	Format	Variable Label
BCFAINHH	1	42-43	F2	CHILD'S FATHER IN SAME HOUSEHOLD?
BCFADIST	1	45-46	F2	DISTANCE OF FATHER FROM CHILD
BCSEEFA	1	48-49	F2	FREQUENCY OF CHILD SEEING FATHER
BCGMINHH	1	51-52	F2	CHILD'S GRANDMOTHER IN SAME HOUSEHOLD?
BCGFINHH	1	54-55	F2	CHILD'S GRANDFATHER IN SAME HOUSEHOLD?
BC1STCC	1	57-58	F2	REGULAR CHILD CARE DURING 1ST YEAR?
BC2NDCC	1	60-61	F2	REGULAR CHILD CARE DURING 2ND YEAR?
BC3RDCC	1	63-64	F2	REGULAR CHILD CARE DURING 3RD YEAR?

BACKGROUND CHARACTERISTICS OF MOTHER (BM)

Variable	Record	Columns	Format	Variable Label
BMBIRTMO	1	66-67	F2	BIRTH MONTH OF MOTHER
BMBIRTYR	1	69-70	F2	BIRTH YEAR OF MOTHER
BMAGE	1	72-73	F2	MOTHER'S AGE IN YRS, TRUNCATED
BMAGE1ST	1	75-76	F2	MOTHER'S AGE AT FIRST BIRTH
BMAFQT80	2	6-9	F4	ARMED FORCES QUALIF TEST SCORE,MOTHR-80
BMMARST	2	11-12	F2	MARITAL STATUS OF MOTHER
BMMARBMO	2	14-15	F2	MONTH 1ST MARRIAGE OF MOTHER BEGAN
BMMARBYR	2	17-18	F2	YEAR 1ST MARRIAGE OF MOTHER BEGAN
BMMAREMO	2	20-21	F2	MONTH 1ST MARRIAGE OF MOTHER ENDED
BMMAREYR	2	23-24	F2	YEAR 1ST MARRIAGE OF MOTHER ENDED
BMONWELF	2	26-27	F2	MOTHER RECEIVED WELFARE PRIOR YR (1985)?
BMWELDOL	2	29-33	F4	AMOUNT OF WELFARE RECD PRIOR YR (1985)
BMFAMINC	2	35-40	F6	TOTAL FAMILY INCOME PRIOR YEAR (1985)
BMPOVERT	2	42-43	F2	FAMILY BELOW POVERTY PRIOR YR (1985)?
BMEMPST	2	45-46	F2	EMPLOYMENT STATUS OF MOTHER
BMHRSWK	2	48-49	F2	# OF HOURS MOTHER WORKED PREVIOUS WEEK
BMLEFTWK	2	51-53	F3	# WKS BEFORE CHILD BORN MOTHER LEFT WORK
BMRETWK	2	55-57	F3	# WKS AFT CHILD BORN MOTHER RETD TO WORK
BMAGEYNG	2	59-60	F2	AGE OF MOTHER'S YOUNGEST CHILD, IN YEARS
BMAGEMEN	2	62-63	F2	MOTHER'S AGE AT MENARCHE
BMAGEINT	2	65-66	F2	MOTHER'S AGE AT FIRST INTERCOURSE
BMHIGRAD	2	68-69	F2	MOTHER'S HIGHEST GRADE COMPLETED
BMASP79	2	71-72	F2	MOTHER'S EDUCATIONAL ASPIRATIONS-79 INT
BMSUSP80	2	74-75	F2	# OF SCHOOL SUSPENSIONS, MOTHER-80 INT
BMEXPL80	3	6-7	F2	# OF SCHOOL EXPULSIONS, MOTHER-80 INT
BMSE80	3	9-10	F2	SELF-ESTEEM SCORE, MOTHER-80 INTERVIEW
BMLOC79	3	12-13	F2	LOCUS OF CONTROL SCORE, MOTHER-79 INT
BMTRAD79	3	15-16	F2	TRADITNL GENDR ROLES SCORE, MOTHR-79 INT
BMSHY85	3	18-19	F2	SELF-RATING OF SHYNESS, MOTHER-85 INT
BMREL79	3	21-22	F2	FREQ OF RELIGIOUS ATTENDNC, MOTHR-79 INT
BMRELYNG	3	24-25	F2	RELIGION MOTHER WAS RAISED IN
BMIDFS79	3	27-28	F2	IDEAL FAM SIZE (# OF KIDS), MOTHR-79 INT
BMDEFS79	3	30-31	F2	DESIRED FAM SIZE (# OF KIDS),MOTH-79 INT

CHILD DEVELOPMENT OUTCOME VARIABLES (CD)

Variable	Record	Columns	Format	Variable Label
CDHOMET	3	33-35	F3	HOME ENVIRONMENT TOTAL STANDARD SCORE
CDHOMECS	3	37-39	F3	HOME ENV-COGN STIMULATION STANDARD SCORE
CDHOMEES	3	41-43	F3	HOME ENV-EMOTIONAL SUPPORT STANDRD SCORE
CDMOTOR	3	45-47	F3	MOTOR & SOCIAL DEVELOPMT STANDARD SCORE
CDBPITOT	3	49-51	F3	BEHAVIOR PROB INDEX TOTAL STANDARD SCORE
CDBPIANT	3	53-55	F3	BEHAV PROB-ANTISOCIAL STANDARD SCORE
CDBPIANX	3	57-59	F3	BEHAV PROB-ANXIOUS-DEPRESSED STAND SCORE
CDBPIHED	3	61-63	F3	BEHAV PROB-HEADSTRONG STANDARD SCORE
CDBPIHYP	3	65-67	F3	BEHAV PROB-HYPERACTIVE STANDARD SCORE
CDBPIDEP	3	69-71	F3	BEHAV PROB-DEPENDENT STANDARD SCORE
CDBPICON	3	73-75	F3	BEHAV PROB-PEER CONFLICTS STANDARD SCORE
CDSHY	4	6-7	F2	SHYNESS-ANXIETY OF CHILD,INTRVIEWR RATNG
CDBODYP	4	9-10	F2	KNOWLEDGE OF BODY PARTS RAW SCORE
CDMEMLOC	4	12-13	F2	MEMORY FOR LOCATION RAW SCORE
CDMEMWOR	4	15-17	F3	VERBAL MEMORY-WORDS STANDARD SCORE
CDMEMSTO	4	19-21	F3	VERBAL MEMORY-STORY STANDARD SCORE
CDPIATM	4	23-25	F3	PEABODY INDV ASSMT TST-MATH STANDRD SCOR
CDPIATRR	4	27-29	F3	PEAB INDV ASSMT TST-READING RECOG ST SCR
CDPIATRC	4	31-33	F3	PEAB INDV ASSMT TST-READING COMPR ST SCR
CDPPVT	4	35-37	F3	PEAB PICTURE VOCABULARY TEST STAND SCORE

HEALTH OF CHILD VARIABLES (HL)

Variable	Record	Columns	Format	Variable Label
HLDOC1ST	4	39-40	F2	CHILD TAKEN TO DOCTOR FOR ILLNESS YR 1?
HLMAINIL	4	42-43	F2	1ST MAIN ILLNESS REQUIRING DOCTOR YR 1
HLAGEILL	4	45-46	F2	# MOS OLD-1ST TAKN TO DOC FOR ILLNS YR 1
HLNVISIT	4	48-49	F2	# VISITS TO DOCTOR FOR MAIN ILLNESS YR 1
HLHOSP	4	51-52	F2	CHILD ADMITTED TO HOSP FOR ILLNESS YR 1
HLWELBAB	4	54-55	F2	CHILD TAKN FOR WELL-BABY CARE IN 1ST YR?
HLDPT1	4	57-58	F2	CHILD HAD 1ST SET DPT-ORL POLIO IMMUNIZ?
HLDPT2	4	60-61	F2	CHILD HAD 2ND SET DPT-ORL POLIO IMMUNIZ?
HLDPT3	4	63-64	F2	CHILD HAD 3RD SET DPT-ORL POLIO IMMUNIZ?
HLMEASLE	4	66-67	F2	CHILD HAD MEASLES SHOT?
HLBRFED	4	69-70	F2	WAS CHILD BREASTFED?
HLBFEND	4	72-74	F3	# OF WKS OLD WHEN BREASTFEEDING ENDED
HLFORMB	5	6-8	F3	# OF WKS OLD WHEN FORMULA FEEDING BEGAN
HLFORME	5	10-12	F3	# OF WKS OLD WHEN FORMULA FEEDING ENDED
HLMILK	5	14-16	F3	# OF WKS OLD WHEN CHILD BEGAN COW'S MILK
HLSOLIDS	5	18-20	F3	# OF WKS OLD WHEN CHILD BEGAN SOLID FOOD
HLLIMITS	5	22-23	F2	CHILD HAS HLTH CONDTN THAT LIMITS PLAY?
HLMEDREQ	5	25-26	F2	CHILD HAS HLTH CONDTN REQUIRNG MED ATTN?
HLINJURY	5	28-29	F2	# OF INJURIES PAST YR REQUIRNG MED ATTN
HLILLPYR	5	31-32	F2	# OF ILLNSS PAST YR REQUIRING MED ATTN

Variable	Record	Columns	Format	Variable Label
HLCHCKUP	5	34-35	F2	CHILD LAST SAW DOCTOR FOR CHECKUP:
HLDENTIS	5	37-38	F2	CHILD LAST SAW DENTIST FOR CHECKUP:
HLPRVINS	5	40-41	F2	CHILD COVERED BY PRIVATE HLTH INSURANCE?
HLMEDCAD	5	43-44	F2	CHILD'S HEALTH CARE COVERED BY MEDICAID?
HLPSYCH	5	46-47	F2	CHILD SEEN BY PSYCH/COUNSELOR PAST YR?
HLEMPROB	5	49-50	F2	CHILD REFRD FOR EMOTIONAL PROB PAST YR?
HLHEIGHT	5	52-53	F2	CHILD'S HEIGHT IN INCHES
HLWEIGHT	5	55-56	F3	CHILD'S WEIGHT IN POUNDS

MOTHER'S DRUG USE (MD)

Variable	Record	Columns	Format	Variable Label
MDALC83	5	58-59	F2	MOTHER EVER DRINK ALCOHOL? 83 INT
MDALCAGE	5	61-62	F2	AGE MOTHER BEGN DRINKING ALC 1+ PER MO
MDCIG84	5	64-65	F2	MOTHER EVER SMOKE A CIGARETTE? 84 INT
MDCIGAGE	5	67-68	F2	AGE MOTHER 1ST TRIED A CIGARETTE
MDMAR84	5	70-71	F2	MOTHER EVER TRIED MARIJUANA? 84 INT
MDMARAGE	5	73-74	F2	AGE MOTHER 1ST TRIED MARIJUANA
MDAMP84	5	76-77	F2	MOTHER EVER TRIED AMPHETAMINES? 84 INT
MDAMPAGE	6	6-7	F2	AGE MOTHER 1ST TRIED AMPHETAMINES
MDBAR84	6	9-10	F2	MOTHER EVER TRIED BARBITURATES? 84 INT
MDBARAGE	6	12-13	F2	AGE MOTHER 1ST TRIED BARBITURATES
MDTRQ84	6	15-16	F2	MOTHER EVER TRIED TRANQUILIZERS 84 INT
MDTRQAGE	6	18-19	F2	AGE MOTHER 1ST TRIED TRANQUILIZERS
MDLSD84	6	21-22	F2	MOTHER EVER TRIED PSYCHEDELICS 84 INT
MDLSDAGE	6	24-25	F2	AGE MOTHER 1ST TRIED PSYCHEDELICS
MDCOC84	6	27-28	F2	MOTHER EVER TRIED COCAINE 84 INT
MDCOCAGE	6	30-31	F2	AGE MOTHER 1ST TRIED COCAINE

PREGNANCY-RELATED VARIABLES—CHILD'S PREGNANCY (PR)

Variable	Record	Columns	Format	Variable Label
PRCARE	6	33-34	F2	DID MOTHER HAVE ANY PRENATAL CARE?
PRMOCARE	6	36-37	F2	MONTH OF PREGNANCY PRENATAL CARE BEGAN
PRTRIM1	6	39-40	F2	ANY PRENATAL CARE 1ST TRIMESTER?
PRALCUSE	6	42-43	F2	FREQ OF ALC USE BY MOTHER DURING PREG
PRSMOKE	6	45-46	F2	AMNT OF SMOKING BY MOTHER DURING PREG
PRSONOGR	6	48-49	F2	SONOGRAM DONE DURING PREGNANCY?
PRVITAMN	6	51-52	F2	MOTHER TOOK VITAMINS DURING PREGNANCY?

Variable	Record	Columns	Format	Variable Label
PRCALORI	6	54-55	F2	MOTHER REDUCED CALORIES DURING PREG?
PRSALT	6	57-58	F2	MOTHER REDUCED SALT DURING PREGNANCY?
PRDIURET	6	60-61	F2	MOTHER USED DIURETIC DURING PREGNANCY?
PRREDSMO	6	63-64	F2	MOTHER REDUCED SMOKING DURING PREG?
PRREDALC	6	66-67	F2	MOTHER REDUCED ALCOHOL DURING PREG?
PRWTBEF	6	69-71	F3	WEIGHT OF MOTHER BEFORE PREG (POUNDS)
PRWTGAIN	6	73-74	F2	# OF POUNDS GAINED BY MOTHER DURING PREG
PRGESTAT	6	76-77	F2	LENGTH OF GESTATION IN WEEKS
PRCESAR	7	6-7	F2	WAS CHILD DELIVERED BY CESAREAN?
PRBWT	7	9-11	F3	CHILD'S BIRTH WEIGHT (OUNCES)
PRBLENG	7	13-14	F2	CHILD'S LENGTH AT BIRTH (INCHES)
PRMHOSP	7	16-17	F2	# OF DAYS MOTHER IN HOSP AT CHILDBIRTH
PRCHOSP	7	19-21	F3	# OF DAYS CHILD IN HOSPITAL AT BIRTH

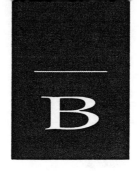

Detailed Description of NLSY Variables

This appendix provides detailed information on the 138 variables in the NLSY extract data set, listed in their order of appearance in the file. **Wherever possible, the actual wording of the question and the response alternatives are provided, indicated with an asterisk (*).** Variables not marked with an asterisk are variables that were constructed from other variables (e.g., a total scale score constructed from 10 individual items). For any questions in which the focal Child is designated as CHILD (all capital letters), the interviewer substituted the focal Child's actual name when asking the questions.

The codes used for response alternatives are also included in this appendix. For uncoded variables (e.g., mother's age at menarche), the range of actual data values for the extract sample is shown.

This appendix also indicates the survey year in which the questions were asked. **If no year is shown, the variable was measured in 1986**—*except* those questions (marked with a † or ‡) that were asked in varying years in relation to the birth date of the focal Child (e.g., information on the focal Child's birth weight was asked in the survey year following the Child's birth) or the mother's marital history.

Variable Name	Description
ADID	Arbitrary identification number assigned to each case, from ID #1001 to 3771. (*Note:* this ID number is *not* the same as the ID number assigned to the case in the full NLSY data set.)
ADINTMO	Month in which the 1986 interview took place:

2	February
3	March
4	April
5	May
6	June
7	July

Variable Name	Description
ADINTYR	Year in which the 1986 interview took place:

Always 86

Variable Name	Description
BCRACE	Race/ethnicity of Child:

1	Hispanic
2	African American
3	Non-Hispanic/non-African American

Variable Name	Description
BCGENDER	Gender of Child

1	Male
2	Female

Variable Name	Description
BCBIRTMO	Month of birth of Child:

1	January
2	February
3	March
4	April
5	May
6	June
7	July
8	August
9	September
10	October
11	November
12	December

Variable Name	Description
BCBIRTYR	Year of birth of Child:

80	1980
81	1981
82	1982
83	1983
84	1984
85	1985
86	1986

Variable Name	Description
BCAGEMON	Child's age in 1986, rounded to the nearest month:

0-71	Actual age in months

Variable Name	Description
BCAGE	Child's age in years in 1986, truncated (i.e., a Child who was 5.5 years old would have a value of 5 for this variable):

0-5	Actual age in years

Variable Name	Description
BCGRADE	Child's current grade in school, 1986:

0	Kindergarten
1	First grade
2	Second grade

Variable Name	Description

BCSPACNG   Spacing (number of months) between Child and next younger sibling, as of 1986 interview:

0	No younger sibling
1-68	Actual number of months

BCHHSIZE   Total number of people residing in same household as Child in 1986, including Child and his/her mother:

2-15	Actual number of household members

BCNSIBS   Total number of siblings of Child residing in the same household as Child in 1986:

0-3	Actual number of siblings

BCFAINHH   *Does CHILD's natural father live in this household?

0	No
1	Yes

BCFADIST   *About how far from you does CHILD's father live?

0	Lives in the same household
1	Within 1 mile
2	1 to 10 miles
3	11 to 100 miles
4	101 to 200 miles
5	More than 200 miles

BCSEEFA   *In the past 12 months (or since CHILD has been separated from his/her father, whichever is most recent), about how often has CHILD seen his/her father?

1	Every day or almost every day
2	2 to 5 times a week
3	About once a week
4	1 to 3 times per month
5	7 to 11 times in the past 12 months
6	2 to 6 times in the past 12 months
7	Once in the past 12 months
8	Never

BCGMINHH   Does Child's grandmother (or step-grandmother) live in the same household as Child in 1986?

0	No
1	Yes

BCGMINHH   Does Child's grandfather (or step-grandfather) live in the same household as Child in 1986?

0	No
1	Yes

BC1STCC   *† In the first year of CHILD's life, was he/she cared for in any *regular* child care arrangement while you worked or participated in some regular activity? (NOTE: This question was not asked of Children who were not yet 1 year old at the time of the interview; if the Child was not yet 1 year of age, the variable is coded as missing.)

0	No
1	Yes

BC2NDCC   *† In the second year of CHILD's life, was he/she cared for in any *regular* child care arrangement while you worked or participated in some regular activity? (NOTE: This question was not asked of Children who were not yet 2 years old at the time of the interview; if the Child was not yet 2 years of age, the variable is coded as missing.)

0	No
1	Yes

*Actual wording of question and response alternatives
† Year of asking this question varies in relation to Child's age

Variable Name	Description		
BC3RDCC	*† In the third year of CHILD's life, was he/she cared for in any *regular* child care arrangement while you worked or participated in some regular activity? (NOTE: This question was not asked of Children who were not yet 3 years old at the time of the interview; if the Child was not yet 3 years of age, the variable is coded as missing.)		
		0	No
		1	Yes
BMBIRTMO	Month of birth of mother of Child:		
		1	January
		2	February
		3	March
		4	April
		5	May
		6	June
		7	July
		8	August
		9	September
		10	October
		11	November
		12	December
BMBIRTYR	Year of birth of mother of Child:		
		57	1957
		58	1958
		59	1959
		60	1960
		61	1961
		62	1962
		63	1963
		64	1964
BMAGE	Mother's age in years in 1986, truncated (i.e., a woman who was 22.8 years old would have a value of 22 for this variable):		
		21-29	Actual age in years
BMAGE1ST	Mother's age in years at the time she first gave birth:		
		15-25	Actual age in years
BMAFQT80	Mother's raw score on the Armed Forces Qualification Test (AFQT), administered in 1980; AFQT scores are a composite of four academic subtests administered as part of the Armed Services Vocational Aptitude Test—word knowledge, paragraph comprehension, arithmetic reasoning, and numerical operations:		
		55-1050	Raw AFQT score
BMMARST	*Just to verify, your current marital status is:		
		1	Never married
		2	Married, or
		3	Separated, divorced, or widowed
BMMARBMO	‡Month in which first marriage of mother began:		
		1	January
		2	February
		3	March

*Actual wording of question and response alternatives
†Year of asking this question varies in relation to Child's age
‡Year of asking question varies in relation to mother's marital history

Variable Name		Description	
		4	April
		5	May
		6	June
		7	July
		8	August
		9	September
		10	October
		11	November
		12	December
		99	Never married
BMMARBYR	‡Year in which first marriage of mother began:		
		75	1975
		76	1976
		77	1977
		78	1978
		79	1979
		80	1980
		81	1981
		82	1982
		83	1983
		84	1984
		85	1985
		86	1986
		99	Never married
BMMAREMO	‡Month in which first marriage of mother ended:		
		1	January
		2	February
		3	March
		4	April
		5	May
		6	June
		7	July
		8	August
		9	September
		10	October
		11	November
		12	December
		98	Still married
		99	Never married
BMMAREYR	‡Year in which first marriage of mother ended:		
		76	1976
		77	1977
		78	1978
		79	1979
		80	1980
		81	1981
		82	1982
		83	1983

‡Year of asking question varies in relation to mother's marital history

Variable Name	Description	
	84	1984
	85	1985
	86	1986
	98	Still married
	99	Never married
BMONWELF	*During 1985, did you (or your husband) receive any payments from Aid to Families with Dependent Children—AFDC?	
	0	No
	1	Yes
BMWELDOL	*During 1985, how much did you (or your husband) receive per month on the average from AFDC? (multiplied times number of months on welfare to yield 1985 annual estimate)	
	0-18,090	Actual dollar amount of AFDC received in 1985
BMFAMINC	Total dollar amount of family income from all sources in the year prior to the 1986 interview (1985):	
	0-160,000	Actual dollar amount of total family income
BMPOVERT	Based on family income and number of household members, was the family below federal poverty guidelines in the year prior to the 1986 interview (1985)?	
	0	No
	1	Yes
BMEMPST	*Now I'd like some information on what you were doing *last week*. What were you doing *most of last week*—working, keeping house, going to school, or something else?	
	1	Working
	2	With a job, but not at work
	3	Looking for work, unemployed
	4	Keeping house
	5	Going to school
	6	Unable to work
	7	Other
	8	Active forces
BMHRSWK	*How many hours did you work *last week* at all jobs (employed women only)?	
	0-90	Actual number of hours worked
BMLEFTWK	Number of weeks before Child was born that mother left employment:	
	0-331	Actual number of weeks
BMRETDWK	Number of weeks after Child was born that mother returned to work:	
	0-100	Actual number of weeks
BMAGEYNG	Age of mother's youngest child at the time of the 1986 interview, in years (truncated):	
	0-6	Actual age in years
BMAGEMEN	*How old were you when you had your first menstrual period? (Asked in 1984)	
	7-18	Actual age in years
BMAGEINT	*How old were you the first time you had sexual intercourse? (Asked in 1984)	
	9-25	Actual age in years
BMHIGRAD	*What is the highest grade or year of regular school that you have completed and gotten credit for?	
	0	No schooling
	1	First grade
	2	Second grade

*Actual wording of question and response alternatives

Variable Name	Description	
	3	Third grade
	4	Fourth grade
	5	Fifth grade
	6	Sixth grade
	7	Seventh grade
	8	Eighth grade
	9	Ninth grade
	10	Tenth grade
	11	Eleventh grade
	12	Twelfth grade
	13	1st year of college
	14	2nd year of college
	15	3rd year of college
	16	4th year of college
	17	5th year of college
	18	6th year of college
	19	7th year of college
	20	8th year of college or more
	95	Ungraded
BMEDASP79	*What is the highest grade or year of *regular* school, that is, elementary school, high school, college, or graduate school, that you would *like* to complete? (Asked in 1979)	
	4	Fourth grade
	5	Fifth grade
	6	Sixth grade
	7	Seventh grade
	8	Eighth grade
	9	Ninth grade
	10	Tenth grade
	11	Eleventh grade
	12	Twelfth grade
	13	1st year of college
	14	2nd year of college (Associate's degree)
	15	3rd year of college
	16	4th year of college (Bachelor's degree)
	17	5th year of college (Master's degree)
	18	More than 5 years of college (Law degree, PhD, MD, LLD, DDS, JD)
BMSUSP80	*Have you ever been suspended from school, even for a short period of time? (IF YES:) Altogether, how many times were you suspended from school? (Asked in 1980)	
	0-50	Actual number of suspensions
BMEXPL80	*Have you ever been expelled from school? (IF YES:) Altogether, how many times were you expelled from school? (Asked in 1980)	
	0-9	Actual number of expulsions
BMSE80	Raw score on Rosenberg's 10-item Self-Esteem Scale; higher scores reflect higher self-esteem. Example of an item: I feel that I'm a person of worth, at least on an equal basis with others—strongly agree / agree / disagree / strongly disagree (scale administered in 1980).	
	24-43	Actual score on scale

*Actual wording of question and response alternatives

Variable Name	Description
BMLOC79	Raw score on a four-item (Rotter) Locus of Control scale. Example of an item—Which is closer to your opinion: What happens to me is my own doing or Sometimes I feel that I don't have enough control over the direction my life is taking? Is the chosen alternative *much closer* or *slightly closer*? Higher scores reflect higher internal orientation—i.e., belief in personal control (scale administered in 1979).
	3-16 Actual score on scale
BMTRAD79	Raw score on an eight-item scale measuring attitudes toward traditional family roles for women. Example of item: A woman's place is in the home, not in the office or shop—strongly agree / agree / disagree /strongly disagree. Higher scores reflect more traditional attitudes about women's family roles (scale administered in 1979).
	8-30 Actual score on scale
BMSHY85	*Thinking about yourself as an adult, would you describe yourself as: (Asked in 1985)
	1 Extremely shy
	2 Somewhat shy
	3 Somewhat outgoing
	4 Extremely outgoing
BMREL79	*In the past year, about how often have you attended religious services—more than once a week, about once a week, two or three times a month, about once a month, several times or less during the year, or not at all? (Asked in 1979)
	1 Not at all
	2 Several times a year or less
	3 About once a month
	4 Two or three times a month
	5 About once a week
	6 More than once a week
BMRELYNG	*In what religion were you raised? (asked in 1979)
	0 No religion
	1 Protestant (no specified denomination)
	2 Baptist
	3 Episcopalian
	4 Lutheran
	5 Methodist
	6 Presbyterian
	7 Catholic
	8 Jewish
	9 Other
BMIDFS79	*Now I'd like to ask you your opinions and expectations about family size. First, what do you think is the ideal number of children for a family? (Asked in 1979)
	0-15 Actual number of children
BMDEFS79	*How many children do *you* want to have? (Asked in 1979)
	0-12 Actual number of children
CDHOMET	Total score on Home Observation for Measurement of the Environment (HOME) Scale—Short Form, age-standardized for the overall sample to have a mean of 100 and a standard deviation of 15 (standardized in 1-year increments). The HOME is a combined maternal report and observational measure of the nature and quality of the Child's home environment. Higher scores reflect more favorable home environments.
	29-133 Age-standardized HOME score

*Actual wording of question and response alternatives

Variable Name	Description
CDHOMECS	Score on the Cognitive Stimulation subscale of the HOME, age-standardized in 1-year increments to have a mean of 100 and a standard deviation of 15. The HOME-CS subscale includes the availability to the Child of books and other enrichment resources and activities. 24-135 Age-standardized subscale score
CDHOMEES	Score on the Emotional Support subscale of the HOME, age-standardized in 1-year increments to have a mean of 100 and a standard deviation of 15. The HOME-ES subscale includes items regarding the mother's warmth and responsiveness to the Child. 50-134 Age-standardized subscale score
CDMOTOR	Standard score on the Motor and Social Development Scale, a 15-item scale that measures milestones in motor, social, and cognitive development in children under age 4, based on the mother's responses to age-appropriate questions; the scale is especially useful for detecting children with developmental delays or handicaps. 59-142 Standard score on scale
CDBPITOT	Standard score on the Behavior Problem Index (BPI), a 28-item scale that measures the frequency, range, and type of childhood behavior problems. The BPI has six subscales measuring different behavioral syndromes in children 4 years of age or older, based on the mother's ratings. Higher scores reflect more behavior problems. 74-143 Standard score on scale
CDBPIANT	Standard score on the Antisocial subscale of the BPI. Example of an item: My child bullies or is cruel or mean to others (not true/sometimes true/often true). 88-140 Standard score on subscale
CDBPIANX	Standard score on the Anxious/Depressed subscale of the BPI. Example of an item: My child feels or complains that no one loves him/her (not true/sometimes true/often true). 86-142 Standard score on subscale
CDBPIHED	Standard score on the Headstrong subscale of the BPI. Example of an item: My child argues too much (not true/sometimes true/often true). 82-126 Standard score on subscale
CDBPIHYP	Standard score on the Hyperactive subscale of the BPI. Example of an item: My child is impulsive, acts without thinking (not true/sometimes true/often true). 86-139 Standard score on subscale
CDBPIDEP	Standard score on the Dependent subscale of the BPI. Example of an item: My child clings to adults (not true/sometimes true/often true). 87-131 Standard score on subscale
CDBPICON	Standard score on the Peer Conflict/Withdrawn subscale of the BPI. Example of an item: My child has trouble getting along with other children (not true/sometimes true/often true). 97-145 Standard score on subscale
CDSHY	*How shy and anxious was CHILD at the end of the Child Supplement? (rating completed by the interviewer) 1-5 Rating from 1 (not at all shy & anxious/sociable & friendly) to 5 (extremely shy, quiet, withdrawn)
CDBODYP	Raw score on the Knowledge of Body Parts Scale, a 10-item measure of the ability of children aged 1 to 2 to identify various parts of their bodies. 0-10 Actual score on scale
CDMEMLOC	Raw score on Memory for Location Scale, a 10-item measure of the ability of children aged 8 months to 3 years 11 months to remember the location of an object that was subsequently hidden from view. 0-10 Actual score on scale

*Actual wording of question and response alternatives

Variable Name	Description
CDMEMWOR	Standard score on Parts A & B (memory for words) of the McCarthy Verbal Memory Scale, a measure of the ability of children aged 3½ through 6 years 11 months to remember words and sentences spoken by the interviewer.
	25-155 Standard score on scale
CDMEMWOR	Standard score on Part C of the McCarthy Verbal Memory Scale, a measure of the ability of children aged 3½ through 6 years 11 months to remember major concepts from a short story read by the interviewer.
	67-155 Standard score on scale
CDPIATM	Standard score on the Mathematics subtest of the Peabody Individual Achievement Test (PIAT), for children aged 5 or older. The subtest measures mathematical skill as taught in mainstream education.
	69-135 Standard score on subtest
CDPIATRR	Standard score on the Reading Recognition subtest of the Peabody Individual Achievement Test (PIAT), for children aged 5 or older. The subtest measures word recognition and pronunciation ability.
	74-135 Standard score on subtest
CDPIATRC	Standard score on the Reading Comprehension subtest of the Peabody Individual Achievement Test (PIAT), for children aged five or older whose raw score on the PIAT Reading Recognition subtest was 19 or higher. The subtest measures the ability to derive meaning from sentences that are read silently.
	95-135 Standard score on subtest
CDPPVT	Standard score on the Peabody Picture Vocabulary Test (PPVT), a scale that measure a child's receptive (hearing) vocabulary of words presented orally by the interviewer, for children age 3 and older.
	41-147 Standard score on test
HLDOC1ST	*†In CHILD's first year, did you take him/her to a clinic, hospital, or doctor because he/she was sick or injured?
	0 No
	1 Yes
HLMAINIL	*†When you took CHILD to a clinic, hospital, or doctor the first time because he/she was sick or injured, what was the nature of his/her illness or injury? (IF MORE THAN ONE MENTIONED, PROBE: What was the main illness or injury?)
	0 None—no illness or injury first year
	1 Fever
	2 Cold
	3 Sore throat
	4 Pneumonia
	5 Ear infection
	6 Vomiting-diarrhea
	7 Rash
	8 Accident-poisoning
	9 Convulsions
	10 Jaundice
	11 Feeding problems
	12 Meningitis
	13 Asthma-bronchitis
	14 Other
HLAGEILL	*†How many months old was CHILD when you took him/her to a clinic, hospital, or doctor the first time for this illness/injury?
	01-12 Actual number of months
HLNVISIT	*†In CHILD's first year, altogether how many visits were made to a clinic, hospital, or doctor because he/she had (ILLNESS)?
	0-40 Actual number of visits

*Actual wording of question and response alternatives
†Year of asking this question varies in relation to Child's age

Variable Name	Description
HLHOSP	*†When CHILD was taken for care because he/she had (ILLNESS), was CHILD admitted to the hospital? 0 No 1 Yes
HLWELBAB	*†In CHILD's first year, did you take him/her to a clinic or doctor for well baby care when he/she was *not* sick? 0 No 1 Yes
HLDPT1	*†Children are given a series of DPT shots (that is, diphtheria, pertussis, tetanus) and oral polio vaccine during the first year of life. We would like to ask some questions about DPT shots for CHILD. Has CHILD had the first set of immunizations, often given when 2 months old? 0 No 1 Yes
HLDPT2	*†Has CHILD had the second set of immunizations, often given when 4 months old? 0 No 1 Yes
HLDPT3	*†Has CHILD had the third set of immunizations, often given when 6 months old? 0 No 1 Yes
HLMEASLE	*†Babies often get a measles shot when they are a little older. Has CHILD had a measles shot? 0 No 1 Yes
HLBRFED	*†When CHILD was an infant, did you breastfeed him/her at all? 0 No 1 Yes
HLBFEND	*†(IF YES:) How many weeks old was he/she when you quit breastfeeding him/her altogether? 0 Still breastfeeding 1-104 Actual number of weeks
HLFORMB	*†How many weeks old was CHILD when you began feeding him/her formula on a daily basis? 0 From birth 1-48 Actual number of weeks 995 Did not formula feed
HLFORME	*†How many weeks old was CHILD when you stopped feeding him/her formula on a daily basis? 0 Still formula feeding 1-398 Actual number of weeks
HLMILK	*†How many weeks old was CHILD when he/she began drinking cow's milk on a daily basis? 0 From birth 1-96 Actual number of weeks 995 Has not begun yet
HLSOLIDS	*†Now we would like you to think about solid food. Solid food is any food other than milk or formula, like cereal or fruit, whether it is commercially prepared like Gerbers, or prepared at home. How many weeks old was CHILD when he/she first ate solid food on a daily basis? 0 From birth 1-76 Actual number of weeks 995 Has not begun yet
HLLIMITS	*Does CHILD have any physical, emotional, or mental condition that limits or prevents his/her ability to do usual childhood activities such as play or participate in games or sports? 0 No 1 Yes

*Actual wording of question and response alternatives
†Year of asking this question varies in relation to Child's age

Variable Name	Description
HLMEDREQ	*Does CHILD have any physical, emotional, or mental condition that requires frequent attention or treatment from a doctor or other health professional?
	0 No
	1 Yes
HLINJURY	*During the past 12 months, has CHILD had any accidents or injuries that required medical attention? (IF YES:) How many such accidents or injuries has CHILD had in the past 12 months?
	0-12 Actual number of accidents or injuries
HLILLPYR	*During the past 12 months, has CHILD had any illnesses that required medical attention or treatment? (IF YES:) How many such illnesses has CHILD had in the past 12 months?
	0-50 Actual number of illnesses
HLCHCKUP	*When did CHILD last see a doctor for a routine health checkup?
	1 Less than 1 month ago
	2 1-3 months ago
	3 4-6 months ago
	4 7-11 months ago
	5 1 year to 23 months ago
	6 2 or more years ago
	7 Never
HLDENTIS	*When did CHILD last see a dentist for a checkup or to have some dental work done?
	1 Less than 1 month ago
	2 1-3 months ago
	3 4-6 months ago
	4 7-11 months ago
	5 1 year to 23 months ago
	6 2 or more years ago
	7 Never
HLPRVINS	*Is CHILD's health care now covered by health insurance provided either by an employer or by an individual plan that pays part or all of a hospital, doctor's, or surgeon's bill?
	0 No
	1 Yes
HLMEDCAD	*There is a national program called Medicaid that pays for health care for persons in need. Is CHILD's health care now covered by Medicaid?
	0 No
	1 Yes
HLPSYCH	*(IF CHILD IS 3 OR OLDER:) During the past 12 months has CHILD seen a psychiatrist, psychologist, counselor, or therapist about any behavioral, emotional or mental problems?
	0 No
	1 Yes
HLEMPROB	*During the past 12 months, have you felt, or has anyone suggested, that CHILD needed help for any behavioral, emotional, or mental problem?
	0 No
	1 Yes
HLHEIGHT	Child's height, in inches, 1986 (measured by interviewer):
	13-59 Actual height in inches
HLWEIGHT	Child's weight, in pounds, 1986 (measured by interviewer):
	7-92 Actual weight in pounds

*Actual wording of question and response alternatives

Variable Name	Description
MDALC83	*Next I'd like to ask you some questions about drinking alcoholic beverages, including beer, wine, and liquor. Have you ever had a drink of an alcoholic beverage? (asked in 1983) 0 No 1 Yes
MDALCAGE	*(IF YES:) How old were you when you first began drinking alcoholic beverages on a regular basis, that is, at least once or twice a month? (asked in 1983) 0 Do not drink once or twice a month 6-23 Actual age in years
MDCIG84	Has mother ever tried a cigarette? (Asked in 1984) 0 No 1 Yes
MDCIGAGE	*(IF YES:) About how old were you when you first tried a cigarette? (Asked in 1984) 3-23 Actual age in years
MDMAR84	Has mother ever used marijuana or hashish? (Asked in 1984) 0 No 1 Yes
MDMARAGE	*(IF YES:) When did you use marijuana or hashish for the first time? How old were you then? (Asked in 1984) 8-24 Actual age in years
MDAMP84	*Please look at this card. Have you *ever* used any of these drugs on your own, without a doctor telling you to take them, to get high or enjoy the feeling? These include amphetamines or stimulants, like uppers, speed, bennies, or diet pills. (Asked in 1984) 0 No 1 Yes
MDAMPAGE	*(IF YES:) How old were you the first time you used an amphetamine or stimulant on your own, without a doctor telling you to take it? (Asked in 1984) 13-25 Actual age in years
MDBAR84	*Have you *ever* used...barbiturates or sedatives on your own, like downers, reds, yellows, quaaludes, or seconal? (Asked in 1984) 0 No 1 Yes
MDBARAGE	*(IF YES:) How old were you the first time you used a barbiturate or sedative on your own, without a doctor telling you to take it? (Asked in 1984) 12-23 Actual age in years
MDTRQ84	*Have you *ever* used...tranquilizers on your own, like Librium or Valium? (Asked in 1984) 0 No 1 Yes
MDTRQAGE	*(IF YES:) How old were you the first time you used a tranquilizer on your own, without a doctor telling you to take it? (Asked in 1984) 11-25 Actual age in years
MDLSD84	*Have you *ever* used...psychedelics like LSD, PCP, mescaline, peyote, or angel dust? (Asked in 1984) 0 No 1 Yes
MDLSDAGE	*(IF YES:) How old were you the first time you used a psychedelic? (Asked in 1984) 12-23 Actual age in years
MDCOC84	*Have you *ever* used...cocaine? (Asked in 1984) 0 No 1 Yes

*Actual wording of question and response alternatives

Variable Name	Description
MDCOCAGE	*(IF YES:) How old were you the first time you used cocaine? (Asked in 1984) 12-24 Actual age in years
PRCARE	*†During your pregnancy with (CHILD), did you make any visits to a doctor or nurse for prenatal care, that is, to be examined or talk about your pregnancy? 0 No 1 Yes
PRMOCARE	*†(IF YES:) When did you first visit a doctor or nurse for prenatal care—during which month of your pregnancy? 1 First 2 Second 3 Third 4 Fourth 5 Fifth 6 Sixth 7 Seventh 8 Eighth 9 Ninth
PRTRIM1	Did prenatal care begin in the first trimester of the pregnancy with CHILD? 0 No 1 Yes
PRALCUSE	*†How often did you usually drink alcoholic beverages, including beer, wine, or liquor, during your pregnancy with CHILD? 0 Never 1 Less than once a month 2 About once a month 3 3 or 4 days a month 4 1 or 2 days a week 5 3 or 4 days a week 6 Nearly every day 7 Every day
PRSMOKE	*†On the average, how many cigarettes did you smoke during your pregnancy? 0 Did not smoke during the pregnancy 1 Less than 1 pack a day 2 1 or more but less than 2 packs a day 3 2 or more packs a day
PRSONOGR	*†Ultrasound or sonogram is a way of taking a picture of the baby through sound waves while the baby is still in the womb. Did you have this test done when you were pregnant with CHILD? 0 No 1 Yes
PRVITAMN	*†During your pregnancy, did you take a vitamin or mineral supplement? 0 No 1 Yes
PRCALORI	*†During your pregnancy, did you cut down on the amount of calories in the food you ate? 0 No 1 Yes

*Actual wording of question and response alternatives
†Year of asking this question varies in relation to Child's age

Variable Name	Description
PRSALT	*†During your pregnancy, did you cut down on the amount of salt you used?
	0 No
	1 Yes
PRDIURET	*†During your pregnancy, did you use diuretics (fluid or water pills) to help eliminate water?
	0 No
	1 Yes
PRREDSMO	*†During your pregnancy, did you reduce or stop your smoking?
	0 No
	1 Yes
	4 Not applicable
PRREDALC	*†During your pregnancy, did you reduce or stop your alcohol intake?
	0 No
	1 Yes
	4 Not applicable
PRWTBEF	*†What was your weight just before you became pregnant with CHILD?
	67-324 Actual weight in pounds
PRWTGAIN	Number of pounds gained during pregnancy (subtraction of response to PRWTBEF from response to following: "What was your weight just before you delivered?"):
	0-96 Actual number of pounds gained
PRGESTAT	Length of gestational period in weeks:
	13-47 Actual number of weeks
PRCESAR	*†Was a cesarean section done? (PROBE, IF NECESSARY:) Was the baby delivered by incision in your abdomen?
	0 No
	1 Yes
PRBWT	*†How much did CHILD weigh at birth?
	28-174 Actual birth weight in ounces
PRBLENG	*†What was CHILD's length at birth?
	9-48 Actual length, in inches
PRMHOSP	Number of days mother stayed in hospital at birth of Child (Response to PRCHOSP ± response to the question: "How many days earlier/later did you leave the hospital?"):
	0-51 Actual number of days in the hospital
PRCHOSP	*†How long did your baby stay in the hospital?
	0-90 Actual number of days in the hospital

·Actual wording of question and response alternatives
†Year of asking this question varies in relation to Child's age

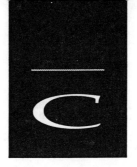

Codebook for NLSY Variables, Listed in Alphabetical Order

```
Variable: ADID          Label: CASE ID NUMBER
   No value labels       Type: Number  Width:  4  Dec: 0      Missing: * None *

Variable: ADINTMO       Label: MONTH OF 1986 INTERVIEW
   Value labels follow   Type: Number  Width:  2  Dec: 0      Missing:   -1.00
       1.00   JANUARY                      2.00   FEBRUARY
       3.00   MARCH                        4.00   APRIL
       5.00   MAY                          6.00   JUNE
       7.00   JULY                         8.00   AUGUST
       9.00   SEPTEMBER                   10.00   OCTOBER
      11.00   NOVEMBER                    12.00   DECEMBER

Variable: ADINTYR       Label: YEAR OF 1986 INTERVIEW
   Value labels follow   Type: Number  Width:  2  Dec: 0      Missing:   -1.00
      86.00   1986

Variable: BCAGE         Label: CHILD'S AGE IN YRS, TRUNCATED
   No value labels       Type: Number  Width:  2  Dec: 0      Missing:   -1.00

Variable: BCAGEMON      Label: CHILD'S AGE IN MONTHS
   No value labels       Type: Number  Width:  2  Dec: 0      Missing:   -1.00

Variable: BCBIRTMO      Label: BIRTH MONTH OF CHILD
   Value labels follow   Type: Number  Width:  2  Dec: 0      Missing:   -1.00
       1.00   JANUARY                      2.00   FEBRUARY
       3.00   MARCH                        4.00   APRIL
       5.00   MAY                          6.00   JUNE
       7.00   JULY                         8.00   AUGUST
       9.00   SEPTEMBER                   10.00   OCTOBER
      11.00   NOVEMBER                    12.00   DECEMBER

Variable: BCBIRTYR      Label: BIRTH YEAR OF CHILD
   Value labels follow   Type: Number  Width:  2  Dec: 0      Missing:   -1.00
      80.00   1980                        81.00   1981
      82.00   1982                        83.00   1983
      84.00   1984                        85.00   1985
      86.00   1986

Variable: BCFADIST      Label: DISTANCE OF FATHER FROM CHILD
   Value labels follow   Type: Number  Width:  2  Dec: 0      Missing:   -1.00
        .00   SAME HOUSE                   1.00   WITHIN 1 MILE
       2.00   1-10 MILES                   3.00   11-100 MILES
       4.00   101-200 MILES                5.00   > 200 MILES

Variable: BCFAINHH      Label: CHILD'S FATHER IN SAME HOUSEHOLD?
   Value labels follow   Type: Number  Width:  2  Dec: 0      Missing:   -1.00
        .00   NO                           1.00   YES

Variable: BCGENDER      Label: GENDER OF CHILD
   Value labels follow   Type: Number  Width:  2  Dec: 0      Missing:   -1.00
       1.00   MALE                         2.00   FEMALE
```

```
Variable: BCGFINHH     Label: CHILD'S GRANDFATHER IN SAME HOUSEHOLD?
   Value labels follow  Type: Number  Width:  2  Dec: 0     Missing:    -1.00
      .00   NO                            1.00   YES

Variable: BCGMINHH     Label: CHILD'S GRANDMOTHER IN SAME HOUSEHOLD?
   Value labels follow  Type: Number  Width:  2  Dec: 0     Missing:    -1.00
      .00   NO                            1.00   YES

Variable: BCGRADE      Label: CHILD'S GRADE IN SCHOOL
   Value labels follow  Type: Number  Width:  2  Dec: 0     Missing:    -1.00
      .00   KINDERGARTEN                  1.00   1ST GRADE
     2.00   2ND GRADE

Variable: BCHHSIZE     Label: # OF HOUSEHOLD MEMBERS
   No value labels      Type: Number  Width:  2  Dec: 0     Missing:    -1.00

Variable: BCNSIBS      Label: # OF CHILD'S SIBLINGS IN SAME HOUSEHOLD
   No value labels      Type: Number  Width:  2  Dec: 0     Missing:    -1.00

Variable: BCRACE       Label: RACE-ETHNICITY OF CHILD
   Value labels follow  Type: Number  Width:  2  Dec: 0     Missing:    -1.00
     1.00   HISPANIC                      2.00   AFRICAN-AMERICAN
     3.00   NONHISP,NON AFR-AMERICAN

Variable: BCSEEFA      Label: FREQUENCY OF CHILD SEEING FATHER
   Value labels follow  Type: Number  Width:  2  Dec: 0     Missing:    -1.00
     1.00   EVERY DAY                     2.00   2-5 TIMES A WK
     3.00   ONCE A WK                     4.00   1-3 TIMES A MONTH
     5.00   7-11 TIMES PAST 12 MO         6.00   2-6 TIMES PAST 12 MO
     7.00   ONCE PAST 12 MONTHS           8.00   NEVER

Variable: BCSPACNG     Label: # MONTHS TO NXT YOUNGER SIBLING OF CHILD
   Value labels follow  Type: Number  Width:  2  Dec: 0     Missing:    -1.00
      .00   NO YOUNGER SIB

Variable: BC1STCC      Label: REGULAR CHILD CARE DURING 1ST YEAR?
   Value labels follow  Type: Number  Width:  2  Dec: 0     Missing:    -1.00
      .00   NO                            1.00   YES

Variable: BC2NDCC      Label: REGULAR CHILD CARE DURING 2ND YEAR?
   Value labels follow  Type: Number  Width:  2  Dec: 0     Missing:    -1.00
      .00   NO                            1.00   YES

Variable: BC3RDCC      Label: REGULAR CHILD CARE DURING 3RD YEAR?
   Value labels follow  Type: Number  Width:  2  Dec: 0     Missing:    -1.00
      .00   NO                            1.00   YES

Variable: BMAFQT80     Label: ARMED FORCES QUALIF TEST SCORE, MOTHR-80
   No value labels      Type: Number  Width:  4  Dec: 0     Missing:    -1.00

Variable: BMAGE        Label: MOTHER'S AGE IN YRS, TRUNCATED
   No value labels      Type: Number  Width:  2  Dec: 0     Missing:    -1.00

Variable: BMAGEINT     Label: MOTHER'S AGE AT FIRST INTERCOURSE
   No value labels      Type: Number  Width:  2  Dec: 0     Missing:    -1.00
```

Variable: BMAGEMEN   Label: MOTHER'S AGE AT MENARCHE
No value labels   Type: Number Width: 2 Dec: 0   Missing: -1.00

Variable: BMAGEYNG   Label: AGE OF MOTHER'S YOUNGEST CHILD, IN YEARS
No value labels   Type: Number Width: 2 Dec: 0   Missing: -1.00

Variable: BMAGE1ST   Label: MOTHER'S AGE AT FIRST BIRTH
No value labels   Type: Number Width: 2 Dec: 0   Missing: -1.00

Variable: BMASP79   Label: MOTHER'S EDUCATIONAL ASPIRATIONS-79 INT
Value labels follow   Type: Number Width: 2 Dec: 0   Missing: -1.00
    1.00 · 1ST GRADE   2.00   2ND GRADE
    3.00   3RD GRADE   4.00   4TH GRADE
    5.00   5TH GRADE   6.00   6TH GRADE
    7.00   7TH GRADE   8.00   8TH GRADE
    9.00   9TH GRADE   10.00   10TH GRADE
   11.00   11TH GRADE   12.00   12TH GRADE
   13.00   1ST YR COL   14.00   2ND YR COL
   15.00   3RD YR COL   16.00   4TH YR COL
   17.00   5TH YR COL   18.00   6TH+ YR COL

Variable: BMBIRTMO   Label: BIRTH MONTH OF MOTHER
Value labels follow   Type: Number Width: 2 Dec: 0   Missing: -1.00
    1.00   JANUARY   2.00   FEBRUARY
    3.00   MARCH   4.00   APRIL
    5.00   MAY   6.00   JUNE
    7.00   JULY   8.00   AUGUST
    9.00   SEPTEMBER   10.00   OCTOBER
   11.00   NOVEMBER   12.00   DECEMBER

Variable: BMBIRTYR   Label: BIRTH YEAR OF MOTHER
Value labels follow   Type: Number Width: 2 Dec: 0   Missing: -1.00
   57.00   1957   58.00   1958
   59.00   1959   60.00   1960
   61.00   1961   62.00   1962
   63.00   1963   64.00   1964

Variable: BMDEFS79   Label: DESIRED FAM SIZE (# OF KIDS),MOTH-79 INT
No value labels   Type: Number Width: 2 Dec: 0   Missing: -1.00

Variable: BMEMPST   Label: EMPLOYMENT STATUS OF MOTHER
Value labels follow   Type: Number Width: 2 Dec: 0   Missing: -1.00
    1.00   EMPLOYED   2.00   WITH JOB NOT AT WORK
    3.00   UNEMPLOYED   4.00   KEEPING HOUSE
    5.00   IN SCHOOL   6.00   UNABLE TO WORK
    7.00   OTHER   8.00   ACTIVE FORCES

Variable: BMEXPL80   Label: # OF SCHOOL EXPULSIONS, MOTHER-80 INT
No value labels   Type: Number Width: 2 Dec: 0   Missing: -1.00

Variable: BMFAMINC   Label: TOTAL FAMILY INCOME PRIOR YEAR (1985)
No value labels   Type: Number Width: 6 Dec: 0   Missing: -1.00

Variable: BMHIGRAD   Label: MOTHER'S HIGHEST GRADE COMPLETED
   Value labels follow   Type: Number Width: 2 Dec: 0   Missing: -1.00
        .00   NONE   1.00   1ST GRADE
       2.00   2ND GRADE   3.00   3RD GRADE
       4.00   4TH GRADE   5.00   5TH GRADE
       6.00   6TH GRADE   7.00   7TH GRADE
       8.00   8TH GRADE   9.00   9TH GRADE
      10.00   10TH GRADE   11.00   11TH GRADE
      12.00   12TH GRADE   13.00   1ST YR COL
      14.00   2ND YR COL   15.00   3RD YR COL
      16.00   4TH YR COL   17.00   5TH YR COL
      18.00   6TH YR COL   19.00   7TH YR COL
      20.00   8TH YR COL   95.00   UNGRADED

Variable: BMHRSWK   Label: # OF HOURS MOTHER WORKED PREVIOUS WEEK
   No value labels   Type: Number Width: 2 Dec: 0   Missing: -1.00

Variable: BMIDFS79   Label: IDEAL FAM SIZE (# OF KIDS), MOTHR-79 INT
   No value labels   Type: Number Width: 2 Dec: 0   Missing: -1.00

Variable: BMLEFTWK   Label: # WKS BEFORE CHILD BORN MOTHER LEFT WORK
   No value labels   Type: Number Width: 3 Dec: 0   Missing: -1.00

Variable: BMLOC79   Label: LOCUS OF CONTROL SCORE, MOTHER-79 INT
   No value labels   Type: Number Width: 2 Dec: 0   Missing: -1.00

Variable: BMMARBMO   Label: MONTH 1ST MARRIAGE OF MOTHER BEGAN
   Value labels follow   Type: Number Width: 2 Dec: 0   Missing: -1.00
       1.00   JANUARY   2.00   FEBRUARY
       3.00   MARCH   4.00   APRIL
       5.00   MAY   6.00   JUNE
       7.00   JULY   8.00   AUGUST
       9.00   SEPTEMBER   10.00   OCTOBER
      11.00   NOVEMBER   12.00   DECEMBER
      99.00   NEVER MARRIED

Variable: BMMARBYR   Label: YEAR 1ST MARRIAGE OF MOTHER BEGAN
   Value labels follow   Type: Number Width: 2 Dec: 0   Missing: -1.00
      75.00   1975   76.00   1976
      77.00   1977   78.00   1978
      79.00   1979   80.00   1980
      81.00   1981   82.00   1982
      83.00   1983   84.00   1984
      85.00   1985   86.00   1986
      99.00   NEVER MARRIED

Variable: BMMAREMO   Label: MONTH 1ST MARRIAGE OF MOTHER ENDED
   Value labels follow   Type: Number Width: 2 Dec: 0   Missing: -1.00
       1.00   JANUARY   2.00   FEBRUARY
       3.00   MARCH   4.00   APRIL
       5.00   MAY   6.00   JUNE
       7.00   JULY   8.00   AUGUST
       9.00   SEPTEMBER   10.00   OCTOBER
      11.00   NOVEMBER   12.00   DECEMBER
      98.00   STILL MARRIED   99.00   NEVER MARRIED

Variable: BMMAREYR   Label: YEAR 1ST MARRIAGE OF MOTHER ENDED
    Value labels follow Type: Number Width: 2 Dec: 0   Missing: -1.00
        75.00   1975   76.00   1976
        77.00   1977   78.00   1978
        79.00   1979   80.00   1980
        81.00   1981   82.00   1982
        83.00   1983   84.00   1984
        85.00   1985   86.00   1986
        98.00   STILL MARRIED   99.00   NEVER MARRIED

Variable: BMMARST   Label: MARITAL STATUS OF MOTHER
    Value labels follow Type: Number Width: 2 Dec: 0   Missing: -1.00
        1.00   NEVER MARRIED   2.00   MARRIED, SPOUSE PRESENT
        3.00   OTHER

Variable: BMONWELF   Label: MOTHER RECEIVED WELFARE PRIOR YR (1985)?
    Value labels follow Type: Number Width: 2 Dec: 0   Missing: -1.00
        .00   NO   1.00   YES

Variable: BMPOVERT   Label: FAMILY BELOW POVERTY PRIOR YR (1985)?
    Value labels follow Type: Number Width: 2 Dec: 0   Missing: -1.00
        .00   NO   1.00   YES

Variable: BMRELYNG   Label: RELIGION MOTHER WAS RAISED IN
    Value labels follow Type: Number Width: 2 Dec: 0   Missing: -1.00
        .00   NO RELIGION   1.00   PROTESTANT
        2.00   BAPTIST   3.00   EPISCOPALIAN
        4.00   LUTHERAN   5.00   METHODIST
        6.00   PRESBYTERIAN   7.00   CATHOLIC
        8.00   JEWISH   9.00   OTHER

Variable: BMREL79   Label: FREQ OF RELIGIOUS ATTENDNC, MOTHR-79 INT
    Value labels follow Type: Number Width: 2 Dec: 0   Missing: -1.00
        1.00   NOT AT ALL   2.00   INFREQUENTLY
        3.00   ONCE A MONTH   4.00   2-3 TIMES A MONTH
        5.00   ONCE A WK   6.00   > ONCE A WK

Variable: BMRETWK   Label: # WKS AFT CHILD BORN MOTHER RETD TO WORK
    No value labels   Type: Number Width: 3 Dec: 0   Missing: -1.00

Variable: BMSE80   Label: SELF-ESTEEM SCORE, MOTHER-80 INTERVIEW
    No value labels   Type: Number Width: 2 Dec: 0   Missing: -1.00

Variable: BMSHY85   Label: SELF-RATING OF SHYNESS, MOTHER-85 INT
    Value labels follow Type: Number Width: 2 Dec: 0   Missing: -1.00
        1.00   EXTREMELY SHY   2.00   SOMEWHAT SHY
        3.00   SOMEWHAT OUTGOING   4.00   EXTREMELY OUTGOING

Variable: BMSUSP80   Label: # OF SCHOOL SUSPENSIONS, MOTHER-80 INT
    No value labels   Type: Number Width: 2 Dec: 0   Missing: -1.00

Variable: BMTRAD79   Label: TRADITNL GENDR ROLES SCORE, MOTHR-79 INT
    No value labels   Type: Number Width: 2 Dec: 0   Missing: -1.00

Variable: BMWELDOL   Label: AMOUNT OF WELFARE RECD PRIOR YR (1985)
    No value labels   Type: Number Width: 5 Dec: 0   Missing: -1.00

Variable: CDBODYP   Label: KNOWLEDGE OF BODY PARTS RAW SCORE
    No value labels   Type: Number Width: 2 Dec: 0   Missing: -1.00

Variable: CDBPIANT No value labels	Label: BEHAV PROB-ANTISOCIAL STANDARD SCORE Type: Number Width: 3 Dec: 0 Missing: -1.00
Variable: CDBPIANX No value labels	Label: BEHAV PROB-ANXIOUS-DEPRESSED STAND SCORE Type: Number Width: 3 Dec: 0 Missing: -1.00
Variable: CDBPICON No value labels	Label: BEHAV PROB-PEER CONFLICTS STANDARD SCORE Type: Number Width: 3 Dec: 0 Missing: -1.00
Variable: CDBPIDEP No value labels	Label: BEHAV PROB-DEPENDENT STANDARD SCORE Type: Number Width: 3 Dec: 0 Missing: -1.00
Variable: CDBPIHED No value labels	Label: BEHAV PROB-HEADSTRONG STANDARD SCORE Type: Number Width: 3 Dec: 0 Missing: -1.00
Variable: CDBPIHYP No value labels	Label: BEHAV PROB-HYPERACTIVE STANDARD SCORE Type: Number Width: 3 Dec: 0 Missing: -1.00
Variable: CDBPITOT No value labels	Label: BEHAVIOR PROB INDEX TOTAL STANDARD SCORE Type: Number Width: 3 Dec: 0 Missing: -1.00
Variable: CDHOMECS No value labels	Label: HOME ENV-COGN STIMULATION STANDARD SCORE Type: Number Width: 3 Dec: 0 Missing: -1.00
Variable: CDHOMEES No value labels	Label: HOME ENV-EMOTIONAL SUPPORT STANDRD SCORE Type: Number Width: 3 Dec: 0 Missing: -1.00
Variable: CDHOMET No value labels	Label: HOME ENVIRONMENT TOTAL STANDARD SCORE Type: Number Width: 3 Dec: 0 Missing: -1.00
Variable: CDMEMLOC No value labels	Label: MEMORY FOR LOCATION RAW SCORE Type: Number Width: 2 Dec: 0 Missing: -1.00
Variable: CDMEMSTO No value labels	Label: VERBAL MEMORY-STORY, STANDARD SCORE Type: Number Width: 3 Dec: 0 Missing: -1.00
Variable: CDMEMWOR No value labels	Label: VERBAL MEMORY-WORDS, STANDARD SCORE Type: Number Width: 3 Dec: 0 Missing: -1.00
Variable: CDMOTOR No value labels	Label: MOTOR & SOCIAL DEVELOPMT STANDARD SCORE Type: Number Width: 3 Dec: 0 Missing: -1.00
Variable: CDPIATM No value labels	Label: PEABODY INDV ASSMT TST-MATH STANDRD SCOR Type: Number Width: 3 Dec: 0 Missing: -1.00
Variable: CDPIATRC No value labels	Label: PEAB INDV ASSMT TST-READING COMPR ST SCR Type: Number Width: 3 Dec: 0 Missing: -1.00
Variable: CDPIATRR No value labels	Label: PEAB INDV ASSMT TST-READING RECOG ST SCR Type: Number Width: 3 Dec: 0 Missing: -1.00
Variable: CDPPVT No value labels	Label: PEAB PICTURE VOCABULARY TEST STAND SCORE Type: Number Width: 3 Dec: 0 Missing: -1.00

Variable: CDSHY
  Value labels follow
    1.00   NOT AT ALL
	Label: SHYNESS-ANXIETY OF CHILD,INTRVIEWR RATNG
	Type: Number Width: 2 Dec: 0 Missing: -1.00
	SHY-ANXIOUS 5.00 EXTREMELY SHY-ANXIOUS

Variable: HLAGEILL No value labels	Label: # MOS OLD-1ST TAKN TO DOC FOR ILLNS YR 1 Type: Number Width: 2 Dec: 0 Missing: -1.00

```
Variable: HLBFEND       Label: # OF WEEKS OLD WHEN BREASTFEEDING ENDED
   Value labels follow  Type: Number  Width: 3 Dec: 0     Missing:    -1.00
      .00   STILL BREASTFEEDING

Variable: HLBRFED       Label: WAS CHILD BREASTFED?
   Value labels follow  Type: Number  Width: 2 Dec: 0     Missing:    -1.00
      .00   NO                              1.00   YES

Variable: HLCHCKUP      Label: CHILD LAST SAW DOCTOR FOR CHECKUP:
   Value labels follow  Type: Number  Width: 2 Dec: 0     Missing:    -1.00
      1.00  < 1 MO AGO                      2.00   1-3 MOS AGO
      3.00  4-6 MOS AGO                     4.00   7-11 MOS AGO
      5.00  1 YR-23 MOS AGO                 6.00   2+ YRS AGO
      7.00  NEVER

Variable: HLDENTIS      Label: CHILD LAST SAW DENTIST FOR CHECKUP:
   Value labels follow  Type: Number  Width: 2 Dec: 0     Missing:    -1.00
      1.00  < 1 MO AGO                      2.00   1-3 MOS AGO
      3.00  4-6 MOS AGO                     4.00   7-11 MOS AGO
      5.00  1 YR-23 MOS AGO                 6.00   2+ YRS AGO
      7.00  NEVER

Variable: HLDOC1ST      Label: CHILD TAKEN TO DOCTOR FOR ILLNESS YR 1?
   Value labels follow  Type: Number  Width: 2 Dec: 0     Missing:    -1.00
      .00   NO                              1.00   YES

Variable: HLDPT1        Label: CHILD HAD 1ST SET DPT-ORL POLIO IMMUNIZ?
   Value labels follow  Type: Number  Width: 2 Dec: 0     Missing:    -1.00
      .00   NO                              1.00   YES

Variable: HLDPT2        Label: CHILD HAD 2ND SET DPT-ORL POLIO IMMUNIZ?
   Value labels follow  Type: Number  Width: 2 Dec: 0     Missing:    -1.00
      .00   NO                              1.00   YES

Variable: HLDPT3        Label: CHILD HAD 3RD SET DPT-ORL POLIO IMMUNIZ?
   Value labels follow  Type: Number  Width: 2 Dec: 0     Missing:    -1.00
      .00   NO                              1.00   YES

Variable: HLEMPROB      Label: CHILD REFRD FOR EMOTIONAL PROB PAST YR?
   Value labels follow  Type: Number  Width: 2 Dec: 0     Missing:    -1.00
      .00   NO                              1.00   YES

Variable: HLFORMB       Label: # OF WKS OLD WHEN FORMULA FEEDING BEGAN
   Value labels follow  Type: Number  Width: 3 Dec: 0     Missing:    -1.00
      .00   FROM BIRTH                    995.00   NO FORMULA FEEDING

Variable: HLFORME       Label: # OF WKS OLD WHEN FORMULA FEEDING ENDED
   Value labels follow  Type: Number  Width: 3 Dec: 0     Missing:    -1.00
      .00   STILL FORMULA FEEDNG          995.00   NO FORMULA FEEDING

Variable: HLHEIGHT      Label: CHILD'S HEIGHT IN INCHES
   No value labels      Type: Number  Width: 2 Dec: 0     Missing:    -1.00

Variable: HLHOSP        Label: CHILD ADMITTED TO HOSP FOR ILLNESS YR 1
   Value labels follow  Type: Number  Width: 2 Dec: 0     Missing:    -1.00
      .00   NO                              1.00   YES

Variable: HLILLPYR      Label: # OF ILLNSS PAST YR REQUIRING MED ATTN
   No value labels      Type: Number  Width: 2 Dec: 0     Missing:    -1.00
```

Variable: HLINJURY   Label: # OF INJURIES PAST YR REQUIRNG MED ATTN
  No value labels   Type: Number Width: 2 Dec: 0   Missing: -1.00

Variable: HLLIMITS   Label: CHILD HAS HLTH CONDTN THAT LIMITS PLAY?
  Value labels follow Type: Number Width: 2 Dec: 0   Missing: -1.00
    .00 NO   1.00   YES

Variable: HLMAINIL   Label: 1ST MAIN ILLNESS REQUIRING DOCTOR YR 1
  Value labels follow Type: Number Width: 2 Dec: 0   Missing: -1.00
    .00   NONE   1.00   FEVER
   2.00   COLD   3.00   SORE THROAT
   4.00   PNEUMONIA   5.00   EAR INFECTION
   6.00   VOMIT-DIARRHEA   7.00   RASH
   8.00   ACCIDENT-POISONING 9.00   CONVULSIONS
  10.00   JAUNDICE   11.00   FEEDING PROBLEMS
  12.00   MENINGITIS   13.00   ASTHMA-BRONCHITIS
  14.00   OTHER

Variable: HLMEASLE   Label: CHILD HAD MEASLES SHOT?
  Value labels follow Type: Number Width: 2 Dec: 0   Missing: -1.00
    .00 NO   1.00   YES

Variable: HLMEDCAD   Label: CHILD'S HEALTH CARE COVERED BY MEDICAID?
  Value labels follow Type: Number Width: 2 Dec: 0   Missing: -1.00
    .00 NO   1.00   YES

Variable: HLMEDREQ   Label: CHILD HAS HLTH CONDTN REQUIRNG MED ATTN?
  Value labels follow Type: Number Width: 2 Dec: 0   Missing: -1.00
    .00 NO   1.00   YES

Variable: HLMILK   Label: # OF WKS OLD WHEN CHILD BEGAN COW'S MILK
  Value labels follow Type: Number Width: 3 Dec: 0   Missing: -1.00
    .00   FROM BIRTH   995.00   HAS NOT BEGUN

Variable: HLNVISIT   Label: # VISITS TO DOCTOR FOR MAIN ILLNESS YR 1
  No value labels   Type: Number Width: 2 Dec: 0   Missing: -1.00

Variable: HLPRVINS   Label: CHILD COVERED BY PRIVATE HLTH INSURANCE?
  Value labels follow Type: Number Width: 2 Dec: 0   Missing: -1.00
    .00 NO   1.00   YES

Variable: HLPSYCH   Label: CHILD SEEN BY PSYCH/COUNSELOR PAST YR?
  Value labels follow Type: Number Width: 2 Dec: 0   Missing: -1.00
    .00 NO   1.00   YES

Variable: HLSOLIDS   Label: # OF WKS OLD WHEN CHILD BEGAN SOLID FOOD
  Value labels follow Type: Number Width: 3 Dec: 0   Missing: -1.00
    .00   FROM BIRTH   995.00   HAS NOT BEGUN

Variable: HLWEIGHT   Label: CHILD'S WEIGHT IN POUNDS
  No value labels   Type: Number Width: 2 Dec: 0   Missing: -1.00

Variable: HLWELBAB   Label: CHILD TAKN FOR WELL-BABY CARE IN 1ST YR?
  Value labels follow Type: Number Width: 2 Dec: 0   Missing: -1.00
    .00 NO   1.00   YES

Variable: MDALCAGE   Label: AGE MOTHER BEGN DRINKING ALC 1+ PER MO
  Value labels follow Type: Number Width: 2 Dec: 0   Missing: -1.00
    .00   DONT DRINK 1+ PER MO

```
Variable: MDALC83        Label: MOTHER EVER DRINK ALCOHOL?  83 INT
   Value labels follow   Type: Number  Width:  2  Dec: 0     Missing:    -1.00
        .00   NO                              1.00   YES

Variable: MDAMPAGE       Label: AGE MOTHER 1ST TRIED AMPHETAMINES
   No value labels       Type: Number  Width:  2  Dec: 0     Missing:    -1.00

Variable: MDAMP84        Label: MOTHER EVER TRIED AMPHETAMINES?  84 INT
   Value labels follow   Type: Number  Width:  2  Dec: 0     Missing:    -1.00
        .00   NO                              1.00   YES

Variable: MDBARAGE       Label: AGE MOTHER 1ST TRIED BARBITURATES
   No value labels       Type: Number  Width:  2  Dec: 0     Missing:    -1.00

Variable: MDBAR84        Label: MOTHER EVER TRIED BARBITURATES?  84 INT
   Value labels follow   Type: Number  Width:  2  Dec: 0     Missing:    -1.00
        .00   NO                              1.00   YES

Variable: MDCIGAGE       Label: AGE MOTHER 1ST TRIED A CIGARETTE
   No value labels       Type: Number  Width:  2  Dec: 0     Missing:    -1.00

Variable: MDCIG84        Label: MOTHER EVER SMOKE A CIGARETTE?  84 INT
   Value labels follow   Type: Number  Width:  2  Dec: 0     Missing:    -1.00
        .00   NO                              1.00   YES

Variable: MDCOCAGE       Label: AGE MOTHER 1ST TRIED COCAINE
   No value labels       Type: Number  Width:  2  Dec: 0     Missing:    -1.00

Variable: MDCOC84        Label: MOTHER EVER TRIED COCAINE?  84 INT
   Value labels follow   Type: Number  Width:  2  Dec: 0     Missing:    -1.00
        .00   NO                              1.00   YES

Variable: MDLSDAGE       Label: AGE MOTHER 1ST TRIED PSYCHEDELICS
   No value labels       Type: Number  Width:  2  Dec: 0     Missing:    -1.00

Variable: MDLSD84        Label: MOTHER EVER TRIED PSYCHEDELICS?  84 INT
   Value labels follow   Type: Number  Width:  2  Dec: 0     Missing:    -1.00
        .00   NO                              1.00   YES

Variable: MDMARAGE       Label: AGE MOTHER 1ST TRIED MARIJUANA
   No value labels       Type: Number  Width:  2  Dec: 0     Missing:    -1.00

Variable: MDMAR84        Label: MOTHER EVER TRIED MARIJUANA?  84 INT
   Value labels follow   Type: Number  Width:  2  Dec: 0     Missing:    -1.00
        .00   NO                              1.00   YES

Variable: MDTRQAGE       Label: AGE MOTHER 1ST TRIED TRANQUILIZERS
   No value labels       Type: Number  Width:  2  Dec: 0     Missing:    -1.00

Variable: MDTRQ84        Label: MOTHER EVER TRIED TRANQUILIZERS?  84 INT
   Value labels follow   Type: Number  Width:  2  Dec: 0     Missing:    -1.00
        .00   NO                              1.00   YES

Variable: PRALCUSE       Label: FREQ OF ALC USE BY MOTHER DURING PREG
   Value labels follow   Type: Number  Width:  2  Dec: 0     Missing:    -1.00
        .00   NEVER                           1.00   < ONCE A MONTH
       2.00   ONCE A MONTH                    3.00   3-4 DAYS A MONTH
       4.00   1-2 DAYS A WEEK                 5.00   3-4 DAYS A WEEK
       6.00   NEARLY EVERY DAY                7.00   EVERY DAY
```

```
Variable: PRBLENG          Label: CHILD'S LENGTH AT BIRTH (INCHES)
   No value labels         Type: Number  Width:  2 Dec: 0     Missing:     -1.00

Variable: PRBWT            Label: CHILD'S BIRTH WEIGHT (OUNCES)
   No value labels         Type: Number  Width:  3 Dec: 0     Missing:     -1.00

Variable: PRCALORI         Label: MOTHER REDUCED CALORIES DURING PREG?
   Value labels follow     Type: Number  Width:  2 Dec: 0      Missing:    -1.00
      .00   NO                                     1.00   YES

Variable: PRCARE           Label: DID MOTHER HAVE ANY PRENATAL CARE?
   Value labels follow     Type: Number  Width:  2 Dec: 0      Missing:    -1.00
      .00   NO                                     1.00   YES

Variable: PRCESAR          Label: WAS CHILD DELIVERED BY CESAREAN?
   Value labels follow     Type: Number  Width:  2 Dec: 0      Missing:    -1.00
      .00   NO                                     1.00   YES

Variable: PRCHOSP          Label: # OF DAYS CHILD IN HOSPITAL AT BIRTH
   No value labels         Type: Number  Width:  3 Dec: 0     Missing:     -1.00

Variable: PRDIURET         Label: MOTHER USED DIURETIC DURING PREGNANCY?
   Value labels follow     Type: Number  Width:  2 Dec: 0      Missing:    -1.00
      .00   NO                                     1.00   YES

Variable: PRGESTAT         Label: LENGTH OF GESTATION IN WEEKS
   No value labels         Type: Number  Width:  2 Dec: 0     Missing:     -1.00

Variable: PRMHOSP          Label: # OF DAYS MOTHER IN HOSP AT CHILDBIRTH
   No value labels         Type: Number  Width:  2 Dec: 0     Missing:     -1.00

Variable: PRMOCARE         Label: MONTH OF PREGNANCY PRENATAL CARE BEGAN
   No value labels         Type: Number  Width:  2 Dec: 0     Missing:     -1.00

Variable: PRREDALC         Label: MOTHER REDUCED ALCOHOL DURING PREG?
   Value labels follow     Type: Number  Width:  2 Dec: 0     Missing:     -1.00
      1.00   YES, REDUC ALC                   .00   NO ALC REDUC
      4.00   DO NOT DRINK, NOT APPL

Variable: PRREDSMO         Label: MOTHER REDUCED SMOKING DURING PREG?
   Value labels follow     Type: Number  Width:  2 Dec: 0     Missing:     -1.00
      1.00   YES, REDUC SMOKG                  .00   NO SMOK REDUC
      4.00   DO NOT SMOKE,NOT APPL

Variable: PRSALT           Label: MOTHER REDUCED SALT DURING PREGNANCY?
   Value labels follow     Type: Number  Width:  2 Dec: 0      Missing:    -1.00
      .00   NO                                     1.00   YES

Variable: PRSMOKE          Label: AMNT OF SMOKING BY MOTHER DURING PREG
   Value labels follow     Type: Number  Width:  2 Dec: 0                 -1.00
      .00   DID NOT SMOKE                     1.00   < 1 PACK A DAY
      2.00   1-2 PACKS A DAY                  3.00   2+ PACKS A DAY

Variable: PRSONOGR         Label: SONOGRAM DONE DURING PREGNANCY?
   Value labels follow     Type: Number  Width:  2 Dec: 0      Missing:    -1.00
      .00   NO                                     1.00   YES
```

```
Variable: PRTRIM1        Label: ANY PRENATAL CARE 1ST TRIMESTER?
   Value labels follow   Type: Number  Width:  2  Dec: 0     Missing:     1.00
      .00   NO                                1.00   YES

Variable: PRVITAMN       Label: MOTHER TOOK VITAMINS DURING PREGNANCY?
   Value labels follow   Type: Number  Width:  2  Dec: 0     Missing:    -1.00
      .00   NO                                1.00   YES

Variable: PRWTBEF        Label: WEIGHT OF MOTHER BEFORE PREG (POUNDS)
   No value labels       Type: Number  Width:  3  Dec: 0     Missing:    -1.00

Variable: PRWTGAIN       Label: # OF POUNDS GAINED BY MOTHER DURING PREG
   No value labels       Type: Number  Width:  2  Dec: 0     Missing:    -1.00
```

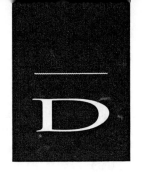

Answers to Selected Exercises

CHAPTER 1

A.1 a. continuous; b. discrete; c. discrete; d. discrete; e. continuous

A.2 a. nominal; b. ratio; c. nominal; d. ratio; e. ordinal

A.4 a. all five of them; b. none of them; c. BCAGEMON, BCAGE; d. 1; e. 3

A.5 a. youngest = age 0; oldest = age 5; b. four; c. 1004, 1007, 1009, 1011; d. 1013; e. 1012 and 1014; these children are not yet 1 year old so all three questions were inapplicable

A.6 a. 1033; b. 15 months; c. 1006; d. three

C.1 a. PREGCNT, LIVEBRTH; theoretically, it is possible for 9 to be a *valid* code for these variables—nine pregnancies and nine live births—and so an out-of-range value had to be used; b. DEPRESS; c. 4; d. 2; e. DEPRESS—the only valid codes are 0, 1, 2, and 9

C.2. a. ID numbers 2, 3, and 7; b. two; c. 2, 6, 12, and 13; d. four; e. 10

CHAPTER 2

A.1 a. 167, 11.6%, 96.2%; b. March, 43.6%; c. July, .3%; d. April; e. 0

A.2 a. 1038 valid cases, 417 missing cases; b. nine; c. 61; d. 58.8%; e. 2%

A.3 Given that the sample for these exercises consists of first-born children who were under age 6, a code of 6 for BMAGEYNG is impossible. The one case coded 6 would have to be examined to determine where the error lies (i.e., is the error at BMAGEYNG, at BCAGE, or at the variable for the Child's birth order, which was used to select cases?).

A.4   784 cases are non-Hispanic, non-African-American

A.5   a. 7%; b. 15 and 16; c. unimodal, fairly symmetric

A.6   a. BCHHSIZE; b. BMASP79; c. BMAGEINT; d. BCHHSIZE

A.7   1182 cases with no missing data

C.1   a. 2106 total cases; b. 791; c. 35.1%; d. 64.9%; e. missing values code = 99; 307 missing cases; 1799 valid cases.

C.2   a. 12, 1 case; b. 35; c. both 40 and 41 have the highest frequency, 130 cases (6%); d. 21 missing cases; e. 5 would be best

C.3   a. 80, 4%; b. twelfth grade, 339 cases; c. bimodal (peaks at eighth and twelfth grade)

CHAPTER 3

A.1   a. mode = 1; b. positively skewed; c. mean would be greater than the mode

A.2   a. mean = 89.4, median = 90.0, mode = 98.0; b. CDMEMWOR and CDPIATRC, because the value of all three indexes are approximately equal; c. negatively, positively, negatively; d. CDPIATRC (1360 missing), CDMEMWOR (616 missing)

A.3   a. range = 106, SD = 18.3, Var = 336.6; b. largest range = CDMEMWOR (130); largest SD = CDPPVT; c. CDPIATM

A.5   a. mean = 4.78, which is not meaningful because BMRELYNG is a nominal-level variable and the numbers are arbitrary codes; b. The mode (7) can be used because it indicates the value with the highest frequency (Catholic).

A.6   a. The value is specified as missing (in SPSS it is ".''—the system missing code) because for this first case CDMEMLOC is coded -1, missing; b. for case 1005, the Z score is (10 7.4) ÷ 3.065 = .848; c. case number 1014 is negative; the raw score is lower than the mean for CDMEMLOC (2.4 SDs below the mean)

A.7   The mean of 608 could be used for mean substitution. Changes following substitution tend to be small (e.g., the mean of 608.276 changes to 608.265; the SD of 199.3 changes to 195.3).

C.1   a. PREGCNT; b. mean pregnancies = 1.893, mean live births = 1.434. c. Both positively skewed, but LIVEBRTH is more skewed (skewness index = 1.517, compared to .784 for PREGCNT); d. all had been pregnant (minimum for PREGCNT = 1.000) but not all had already given birth (minimum for LIVEBRTH = 0.000); e. PREGCNT

C.2   a. 10.0 years old; b. range = 6; c. AGE1BRTH is somewhat more dispersed, but the variability is overall quite similar; d. the program for Figure 3–1 presented descriptive statistics to a higher level of precision—three decimal places versus two.

C.3.   a. yes—the mean of ZCESD is 0 and the SD is 1; b. 0; c. −1.52438; d. 1.00

CHAPTER 4

A.1 a. 127, 193; b. 53.9%, 49.8%; c. 27.9%, 53.2%; d. 54.0%, 51.1%; e. 10.2%, 13.9%, Hispanic girls

A.2 a. 115.7162; b. boys weighed 4.0 ounces more, on average; c. females; d. seven cases with missing values, 0.5% of the sample

A.3 a. strong positive relationship; b. one time (at BCHEIGHT about 39 inches and BCWEIGHT about 30 pounds); c. 46 inches; d. 33 pounds

A.4 a. .9855; b. BCAGEMON and HLHEIGHT; c. height; d. 1432 cases

C.1 a. 1172, 70.9%; b. 608, 36.8%; c. 34.8%, 8.4%; d. 1.2%, 0.4%; e. 452 missing cases, cannot tell from the printout which variable has the missing data

C.2 a. 38.3458, 6.5340; b. 2085 cases, 21 missing cases; c. women with a diploma

C.3 a. DLC, SUPSATIS; b. DLC-ESTEEM; c. CESD, DLC; d. DLC-INTERNAL (.0435)

CHAPTER 5

A.1 a. H_1: $\mu_{PRBWT} \neq 112.0$, H_1: $\mu_{PRBWT} <$ (or >) 112.0; b. H_1: $\mu_{BMAGE1ST}$ 22.0, H_1: $\mu_{BMAGE1ST} <$ (or >) 22.0; c. H_1: $\mu_{BCHHSIZE} \neq 4.0$, H_1: $\mu_{BCHHSIZE} <$ (or >) 4.0

A.2 95% $CI = (12.56 \leq \mu_{MDALCAGE} \leq 13.38)$; 95% $CI = (13.77 \leq \mu_{MDCIGAGE} \leq 14.13)$

A.3 a. outside—an improbable mean age; b. inside—a plausible mean age; c. 95% CI = .36; 99% CI = .46; 99% CI is .10 larger; d. MDALCAGE is larger because the SEM is larger—i.e., age for MDALCAGE is more variable

A.4 a. All null hypothesis are rejected at the .05 level; b. $t = 7.24$; c. 0.00 (all cases have 22 as the value, so there is no variation); d. $df = 1454$

A.5 a. mean = 6.73, $SD = 3.33$; b. $t = 2.59$; c. significant at the .01 level; d. birth months are not randomly distributed; slightly greater tendency for births to occur in the last 6 months of the year, since the mean was greater than 6.5, the midpoint

C.1 a. mean = .4490, $SD = .826$; b. $SEM = .018$, 95% $CI = (.414 \leq \mu_{ABORTS} \leq .484)$; c. $t = 24.91$; d. statistically significant beyond the .001 level (i.e., less than 1 in 1000 chances that the population mean is zero)

C.2 a. 140 white women, 309 nonwhite women; b. whites: 95% $CI = (\$370.82 \leq \mu_{WELF\$MO} \leq \$398.58)$; nonwhites: 95% $CI = (\$389.93 \leq \mu_{WELF\$MO} \leq \$405.93)$; \$395.00 is a plausible average for both whites and nonwhites; c. whites were higher, on average, by \$0.39; d. SEM of HWAGEA was higher for nonwhites, largely because the number of cases was much larger

CHAPTER 6

A.1 a. H_1: $\mu_{PRBWT \text{ for } PRTRIM1(yes)} \neq \mu_{PRBWT \text{ for } PRTRIM1(no)}$; H_1: $\mu_{PRBWT \text{ for } PRTRIM1(yes)} >$ (or <) $\mu_{PRBWT \text{ for } PRTRIM1(no)}$; b. H_1: $\mu_{PRWTGAIN \text{ for } PRCALORI(yes)} \neq \mu_{PRWTGAIN \text{ for } PRCALORI(no)}$; H_1: $\mu_{PRWTGAIN \text{ for } PRCALORI(yes)} >$ (or <) $\mu_{PRWTGAIN \text{ for } PRCALORI(no)}$;

c. H_1: $\mu_{PRGESTAT \text{ for } PRCESAR(yes)} \neq \mu_{PRGESTAT \text{ for } PRCESAR(no)}$; H_1: $\mu_{PRGESTAT \text{ for }}$
$PRCESAR(yes) > (\text{or} <) \mu_{PRGESTAT \text{ for } PRCESAR(no)}$

A.2 a. $t = -2.66$, $t = 2.60$, $t = -1.51$; b. a and b; c. a and b; d. no (for the third hypothesis, a one-tailed test would be significant at about .065); e. none of them; f. (a) The mean birth weight for children whose mothers had first trimester prenatal care (mean = 116.4 ounces) is significantly higher than that for children whose mothers did not receive first trimester prenatal care (mean = 113.1); (b) The mean number of pounds gained during pregnancy is significantly higher for women who did not reduce caloric intake (mean = 34.4 pounds) than for women who did (mean = 32.0 pounds); (c) There is no significant difference in number of weeks of gestation among those infants who were born by cesarean birth (mean = 38.8 weeks) and those who were not (mean = 38.5 weeks).

A.3 a. H_1: $\mu_{BMSUSP80} \neq \mu_{BMEXPL80}$, H_1: $\mu_{BMSUSP80} > (\text{or} <) \mu_{BMEXPL80}$; b. H_1: $\mu_{MDCIGAGE}$ $\neq \mu_{MDALCAGE}$, H_1: $\mu_{MDCIGAGE} > (\text{or} <) \mu_{MDALCAGE}$; c. H_1: $\mu_{BMASP79} \neq \mu_{BMHIGRAD}$; H_1: $\mu_{BMASP79} > (\text{or} <) \mu_{BMHIGRAD}$

A.4 a. $t = 9.19$, $t = 1.77$, $t = 38.70$; b. a and c; c. a and c; d. yes, two-tailed significance for hypothesis b is .077, and one-tailed significance is .0385 which is < .05; e. (a) mean difference = .4528, 95% CI = $(.356 \leq \mu_{diff} \leq .549)$, (b) mean difference = .4083, 95% CI = $(-.044 \leq \mu_{diff} \leq .860)$, (c) mean difference = 2.0415, 95% CI = $(1.938 \leq \mu_{diff} \leq 2.145)$; f. (a) The women had significantly more school suspensions (mean = 0.50) than school expulsions (mean = .05); (b) The women did not differ significantly in the age at which they began to drink regularly (mean = 13.6 years) and at which they first tried a cigarette (mean = 13.9 years); (c) The women achieved significantly fewer years of schooling by 1986 (mean = 12.0 years) than they aspired to in 1979 (mean = 14.0).

C.1 a. 1166 women had a subsequent pregnancy, 940 did not; b. mean for those with a new pregnancy = 21.8937, mean for those without a new pregnancy = 22.3096; c. pooled variance $t = 2.79$, separate variance $t = 2.79$; d. The pooled variance formula is appropriate because Levene's test is nonsignificant, $p = .860$; e. significant at .05 level ($p = .005$); f. Women who had a post-baseline pregnancy had significantly lower mean scores on the Mastery Scale (mean = 21.9) than women who did not have a post-baseline pregnancy (mean = 22.3). g. $r_{pb} = .17$.

C.2 a. 2086 women; b. baseline mean = 18.1088; follow-up mean = 15.9971; c. mean difference = 2.1117, 95% CI = $(1.632 \leq \mu_{diff} \leq 2.592)$; d. $t = 8.63$, $df = 2085$; e. null can be rejected, exact probability is < .001; f. The young mothers scored significantly lower on the depression scale at the follow-up interview (mean = 16.0) than they did 18 months earlier at baseline (mean = 18.1).

CHAPTER 7

A.1 a. no reduction, $n = 165$, reduced smoking, $n = 402$, nonsmokers, $n = 771$; b. highest = nonsmokers (117.4332), lowest = nonreducers (112.8242); c. $MS_B =$

3206.76, $MS_W = 380.62$; d. $F = 8.4251$, $df_B = 2$, $df_W = 1335$; e. yes, significant at the .05 level ($p = .0002$); f. eta$^2 = .0125$ ($6413.5 \div 514542.2$); g. The mothers in the three smoking-habit groups gave birth to infants whose birth weights were significantly different.

A.2 a. All three tests lead to the same conclusion; b. Nonsmokers are significantly different from both smokers who reduced and smokers who did not reduce smoking at the .05 level; c. smokers who reduced smoking are not significantly different from smokers who did not reduce smoking during their pregnancy; d. Infants whose mothers were nonsmokers had mean birth weights (mean = 117.4) that were significantly higher than those of infants whose mothers continued to smoke at pre-pregnancy levels(mean = 112.8) *and* of infants whose mothers reduced smoking during their pregnancies (mean = 113.1); the latter two groups were not statistically different.

A.3 a. 304 Children; b. tallest = African-American, shortest = non-Hispanic, non-African- American; c. $SS_B = 57.2801$, $SS_W = 2289.8219$, $SS_T = 2347.1020$; d. $F = 3.7648$, $df_B = 2$, $df_W = 301$; e. test was significant at .05 level ($p = .0243$); f. African-American Children and non-Hispanic, non-African-American Children; g. African-American Children were significantly taller (mean = 42.6 inches) than Children who were non-Hispanic, non-African-American (mean = 41.6 inches); Hispanic Children (mean = 41.7 inches) were not significantly different from Children in the other two racial/ethnic groups.

A.4 a. Hispanic boys, $n = 35$, African-American girls, $n = 39$; b. tallest = African-American girls (mean = 42.67 inches); shortest = non-Hispanic, non-African-American girls (mean = 41.16 inches); c. $MS_{BCRACE} = 28.957$; $MS_{BCGENDER} = 19.199$; $MS_{Interaction} = 6.214$; d. BCRACE: $F = 3.821$, $df = 2$, 298; BCGENDER: $F = 2.534$; $df = 1$, 298; e. $F = 0.820$, $df = 2$, 298; f. the main effect for BCRACE was statistically significant at the .05 level ($p = .023$)

C.1 a. never received welfare, $n = 749$, always received welfare, $n = 345$; b. never = 17.5251, sometimes = 17.2524, always = 17.0770; c. $MS_B = 28.1685$, $MS_W = 1.9085$; d. $F = 14.7598$, $df = 2$, 2071; e. the null hypothesis can be rejected at the .05 level, p is less than .0001; f. 95% $CI = (17.4301 \leq \mu \leq 17.6200)$, no overlap—the upper value for "always" (17.23) is less than the lower value for "never" (17.43); g. the null hypothesis should be accepted (i.e., variances are homogeneous) because $p > .05$; h. eta$^2 = .014$

C.2 a. difference = .2727; b. all groups are significantly different from each other and so all null hypotheses can be rejected; c. Women who had always been on welfare as a child gave birth at a significantly younger age (mean = 17.1) than women who had never been on welfare (mean = 17.5) or who had been on welfare only occasionally (mean = 17.3). The mean difference for the latter two groups was also statistically significant.

C.3 a. 321, 135, 32; b. highest mean = 17.68, for non-African-Americans never on welfare; lowest mean = 17.05, for non-African-Americans always on welfare *and* African-Americans sometimes on welfare; c. main effect for WELFKID, F = 10.599; main effect for AFR_AMER, F = 32.670; both are statistically significant beyond the .001 level; d. interaction effect, F = 4.338, significant at the .05 level.

C.4 a. 17.296, 16.8551 b. the "always" group; c. between-subjects F = 5.88, significant (p = .003); d. within-subjects F = 69.60, significant (p = .000); e. interaction term F = 0.90, not significant (p = .408)

CHAPTER 8

A.1 a. 126, 22.0%, 55.4%; b. 436, 349.5; c. χ^2 = 120.50111, df = 2; d. the null should be rejected, p < .0001; e. the child's race/ethnicity was significantly related to the likelihood that he or she would be breastfed (χ^2 = 120.5, df = 2, p < .001). African-American children were especially likely not to be breastfed; 22.0% of these children, compared to 45.7% of Hispanic children and 55.7% of non-Hispanic, non-African-American children, were breastfed.

A.2 a. 377 in poverty, 987 not in poverty; b. U = 156097, Z = −3.5647; c. the null hypothesis should be rejected, p = .0004; d. poor women began their prenatal care significantly later into their pregnancies than women who were not poor (U = 156097, p < .001).

A.3 a. 370 never married, 189 other; b. χ^2 = 6.8509 (corrected for ties, 8.3993); c. the null hypothesis can be rejected, p = .0325 (.0150 corrected for ties); d. there was a statistically significant relationship between a woman's marital status and her self-rating of shyness (χ^2 = 8.40, p = .015).

C.1 a. Hospitalization status since baseline and drug use in the past month are independent; b. 157, 15.1%; c. 155, 14.9%; d. 19.4%, 5.1% (19.4% − 14.3%); e. χ^2 = 2.63512 (2.25476 after Yates' correction for continuity); f. null hypothesis cannot be rejected, p = .10452 (.13320 after Yates' correction); g. phi = .05026; h. women who used drugs in the previous month were no more likely to have been hospitalized in the 18 months since baseline than the women who did not (χ^2 = 2.64, df = 1, p > .05).

C.2 a. The population distribution of sick days is the same for the three at-risk groups; b. the at-high-risk group, n = 202; c. χ^2 = 14.0182 uncorrected, 15.3982 corrected; d. the null can be rejected, p = .0005; e. the number of sick days a woman had in the 18 months since baseline was significantly different for those in the three at-risk-for-depression groups (χ^2 = 15.40, p < .001). The number of sick days was highest among those at high risk of depression.

C.3 a. The distribution of marijuana use is the same as the distribution of cocaine use among young mothers; b. 1813, 262; c. Z = −13.1083; d. the null hypothesis can be rejected, p < .0001; e. the use of marijuana among the young mothers was significantly higher than the use of cocaine (Z = −13.11, p < .001).

CHAPTER 9

A.1 a. 12.87 (menarche), 17.43 (intercourse); b. $r = .089$; c. statistically significant, $p = .001$; d. there was a modest but significant tendency for women who started menstruation at a younger age to initiate sexual activity earlier ($r = .09$, $df = 1433$, $p = .001$).

A.2 a. PRBLENG and PRBWT, $r = .4670$, statistically significant, $p < .0005$; b. PRMHOSP and PRBWT, $r = -.0076$, not statistically significant, $p = .780$; c. the lower the infant's birth weight, the longer the infant's stay in the hospital ($r = -.29$, $df = 1367$, $p < .001$), although infant birth weight was unrelated to the mother's length of hospital stay ($r = -.01$, $df = 1367$, NS).

A.3 a. males, $r = .1164$, statistically significant, $p = .002$; b. females, $r = .2252$, statistically significant, $p < .0005$; c. $z_r = .117$ (males), $z_r = .229$ (females); d. $z_{obs} = 2.07$, the correlations are significantly different at $= .05$

A.4 $r_S = .909$; b. statistically significant, $p < .00001$; c. there was a strong tendency for children who lived closer to their fathers to see them more frequently ($r_S = .909$, p < .0001)

A.5 a. $r = .24185$, $r^2 = .05849$; b. standard error of estimate $= 18.99228$; c. $Y' = .309228X + 105.315734$

C.1 a. TRAPPED; b. HARDKID; c. TRAPPED and HARDKID, $r = .2700$; d. TRAPPED and NOTCRY, $r = .1049$; e. all rs are statistically significant at the .001 level

C.2 a. mean $= 100.535$, $SD = 14.99$, the HOME scale has been standardized to a mean of 100 and SD of 15 (values are not exact due to some missing cases); b. dependent (Y) = HOME@TOT, predictor (X) = NKIDS; c. $r = -.21511$, $r^2 = .04637$; d. $Y' = 107.189231\ 3.936308X$; e. 91.44

CHAPTER 10

A.1 a. $R = .28875$, unadjusted $R^2 = .08337$, adjusted $R^2 = .08209$; b. 18.74498 (ounces); c. $F = 65.12531$, significant ($p < .00005$); d. both are significant at $p < .00005$; e. $Y' = 88.684992 + .314174X_1 + .128334X_2$; f. R^2 change $= .0249$

A.2 a. $R = .28961$, $R^2 = .08387$; b. R^2 change $= .00050$, not significant ($p = .3767$), $F = .78181$; c. F decreases from 65.12531 to 43.67086; d. all tolerance levels are above .90, indicating no multicollinearity problems; e. $z_{Y'} = .244781z_{X_1} + .154862z_{X_2} + .022625z_{X_3}$

A.3 Mean $= .686$ (i.e., 68.6% are nonsmokers), $SD = .464$

A.4 a. PRWTGAIN, $R^2 = .05839$; b. NOSMOKE, R^2 change $= .02585$, PRWTBEF has a higher bivariate correlation ($r = .152$) than NOSMOKE ($r = .150$); c. PRWTBEF enters on step 3; d. BMAGE1ST does not enter, $p = .5853$; e. final $R^2 = .10658$ (unadjusted)

C.1 a. $R = .28665$, $R^2 = .08217$ (unadjusted), .08123 (adjusted), the adjustment is small because the sample size is large; b. $F = 87.82154$, statistically significant, $p < .00005$, $df = 2$, 1962; c. $t = -8.760$, statistically significant ($p < .00005$); d. holding number of children constant, for every 1 point increase on the depression scale, the score on the HOME scale is predicted to decrease by .277 points; e. $Y' = 111.359410 - .277301X_1 - 3.807806X_2$

C.2 a. HUSBAND, R^2 change = .01266, $F = 27.42315$; b. NKIDS and CESD; c. predicted increase of 6.33 points on the HOME scale, after controlling NKIDS and CESD; d. about 3.6 times more important (4.60% of variance versus 1.27%); e. ANYDRUG and DIPLOMA, DIPLOMA would enter on the fourth step; f. no multicollinearity problem, all tolerances are in excess of .95

CHAPTER 11

A.1 a. $F = 11.057$, significant, $p = .001$; b. $F = 6.097$, significant, $p = .002$; c. Hispanic mean = 2.609; African-American mean = 2.309; others mean = 2.629; d. African-Americans had the smallest mean desired family size, but we cannot conclude the mean is significantly different from the mean of the other two groups without performing a multiple comparison; e. 1.6% of the variance; f. after controlling the women's attitudes toward traditional gender roles, there were significant racial/ethnic differences in desired family size ($F = 6.10$, $df = 2$, 1414, $p = .002$).

A.2   1418 valid cases; b. Pillai's criterion = .00785, significant ($p = .004$); c. Pillai's criterion = .11330, Wilks' lambda = .88925, both significant at $p < .0005$; d. both dependent variables contributed to the rejection of the null hypothesis (both $p < .0005$); e. the MANCOVA results indicated that even after controlling for traditional gender role attitudes, women in the three racial/ethnic groups had significantly different family size ideals and family size desires ($\lambda = .89$, $p < .001$).

A.3 a. we can reject the null hypothesis, $\lambda = .86917$, $p < .0005$; b. three roots, $R_{c1} = .350$, $R_{c2} = .086$, $R_{c3} = .045$, two roots are significant and used in subsequent analyses; c. PRBWT: $-.964$ on root 1, $-.083$ on root 2; NOSMOKE: $-.536$ on root 1, .791 on root 2; d. highest loading on first root = PRBWT ($-.964$), highest loading on second root = PRGESTAT ($-.900$); e. highest loading on first root = PRWTGAIN ($-.696$), highest loading on second root = NOSMOKE (.798); f. the first root concerns infant size at birth, primarily in terms of birth weight; maternal weight gain is particularly correlated with infant size. The second root primarily concerns the influence of maternal smoking on the length of gestation.

C.1 a. $F = 13.790$, significant, $p < .0005$; b. $F = 13.075$, significant, $p < .0005$; c. mean for not at risk = 24.023, mean for at risk = 23.014, mean for at high risk = 22.284; d. those at high risk had lowest mean adjusted score on MWARMTH, but it cannot be concluded that this group is significantly different from the other two groups; e. the analysis of covariance results indicated that, after con-

trolling for number of children, women in different risk groups had significantly different scores on the Maternal Warmth/Responsiveness scale (F = 13.075,
df = 2, 1977, p < .001); scores were highest in the not-at-risk group and lowest
in the at-high-risk group.

C.2 a. M = 28.41, null hypothesis of homogeneous matrices can be rejected at p =
.005; however, since M is highly sensitive and a significance level of .001 is
sometimes recommended, it can be assumed that the MANCOVA is ade-
quately robust; b. Pillai's criterion = .01399; the relationship between the
composite dependent variable and NKIDS plus DEPRESS is significant (p <
.0005); c. Pillai's criterion = .68714, Wilks' λ = .31295, both are significant
(p < .0005); d. stepdown analysis indicates that level of depression is significantly related to both dependent variables; e. the MANCOVA indicated that,
after controlling for number of children, the mother's level of depression was
significantly related to her score on both the Maternal Warmth/Responsive-
ness scale and the Maternal Control/Punitiveness scale (λ = .32, p < .001);
mothers who were at high risk of clinical depression had the highest mean
scores on the Maternal Control scale and the lowest mean scores on the Maternal Warmth scale.

C.3 a. Pillai's criterion = .13665, significant at p < .0005; b. two roots, R_{c1} = .339,
R_{c2} = .147, 85.6%; c. both roots are significant at p < .0005; = .86582;
d. MCONTROL, .960; MWARMTH, .977; e. TESTSCOR, −.731; CESD,
−.684; f. the mother's cognitive skills (reading abilities and having completed
high school) are especially related to her degree of maternal control/punitive-
ness; the mother's level of depression is especially related to her degree of
maternal warmth and responsiveness.

CHAPTER 12

A.1 a. three factors, accounting for 58.6% of the variance; b. highest communality is
for PRSALT (.65188), lowest communality is for PRVITAMN (.47282); c. first
factor: PRSALT (.78109) and PRCALORI (.78024), second factor: NOALC
(.78453 and .76817), third factor: PRTRIM1 (.71410) and PRVITAMN
(.68345); d. possible names: (1) dietary practices, (2) substance use practices,
(3) health care practices

A.2 Since samples are selected at random for this exercise, the questions cannot be
definitively answered. That is, the analyses you will run will not be based on the
same cases that we have run. In several separate runs, however, we consistent-
ly found three factors, accounting for 58% to 60% of the variance. The pattern
of loadings was essentially the same as obtained in Exercise A.1, and therefore
it appears that the factor structure is stable.

A.3 a. six; b. .223 (PRCALORI and PRSALT), all rs are below .30; c. a factor model
does not appear to be appropriate with these variables.

A.4 a. PRSALT, h^2 = .05820; b. PRTRIM1, h^2 = .00837, very low interrelatedness of all variables in the analysis; c. 18.9%; d. both analyses result in three rotated factors, and the same variables are associated with the three factors; however, the loadings are lower, and in the case of the third factor, the loadings are below what is recommended for factor interpretation (i.e., below .30); e. this factor analysis lends further weight to the conclusion from Exercise A.3 that a factor model is inappropriate for these six variables.

C.1 a. mean = 3.21605, item is worded is the opposite direction from most other items—positively rather than negatively, so the item has to be reversed before scoring; b. item 6 (I felt depressed) has especially high correlations with other items (e.g., r = .64864 with item 18) and item 3 (I felt that I could not shake off the blues even with help from my family or friends) also has high correlations; however, item 7 (I felt that everything I did was an effort) has correlations that are well below average; c. a substantial number of correlations are above .30 and many are even above .40, so the items as a set appear factorable.

C.2 a. highest h^2 = item 18 (.60951); lowest h^2 = item 7 (.09161); b. eigenvalue = 6.77761, three factors greater than 1.0 accounting for 57.6% of the variance; c. three factors based on eigenvalues, three factors with at least 5.0% explained variance, one factor based on scree test because of sharp decline after first factor

C.3 a. 16 items with loadings greater than .30, 13 items clearly associated with factor 1, appears to capture depressed state; b. five items with loadings greater than .30, appears to be measuring happiness, item 7 (I felt that everything I did was an effort) does not seem related to happiness[1]; c. five items with loadings greater than .30, two items clearly associated with factor 3, appears to capture interpersonal relations

C.4 a. 18 items have loadings greater than .30, item 7 appears not to "fit" onto the depression scale; b. negative signs indicate which items have to be reversed prior to scoring the scale; c. with respect to item 7, the item could be reworded to more clearly indicate a negative connotation, it could be dropped, or it could be replaced with a totally new item; (if it were dropped, the standard CES-D cutoff values for defining at-risk categories would have to be changed and revalidated); note, however, that the problem with item 7 may be idiosyncratic to this sample of young mothers.

---

[1] One possible explanation for the item's incongruity is that respondents misinterpreted the item to mean something like "I put effort into things I did," which is a positive statement suggesting high energy levels. If this interpretation is correct, the factor is not so much a "happiness" factor as a "positive affect" factor.

CHAPTER 13

A.1 a. 1392 cases, 617 women, 44.3%; b. 119.3 ounces (breastfed), 112.6 ounces (not breastfed), 54.2% males versus 47.4% females were breastfed; c. lambda = .8153, p <.00005, 18.5% variance accounted for; d. highest loading = BMAFQT80 (.77737), lowest loading = HISPANIC (.03358); e. nonbreastfeeders = −.42435, breastfeeders = .53302; f. 432 women, 70.0%, 67.96%

A.2 a. 675 cases, 296 women breastfed, priors = .56148 (nonbreastfeeders), .43852 (breastfeeders); b. lambda = .8134, $p < .00005$, percentage of variance = 18.7%, different from previous analysis by 0.2%; c. 68.00%, different from previous analysis by 0.4%; d. 717 cases, 68.62%, stable classification results, significantly better than chance

A.3 a. selected = 701, unselected = 754, 675 in the analysis subsample; b. −2 LL = 925.51689 initially, .788.109 after entering independent variables; c. model chi-square = 137.408, $p < .00005$; d. 67.70% of the cases correctly classified, marginally lower (0.3%) than with same subsample using discriminant analysis, 68.76% with crossvalidation subsample; e. older mothers significantly *more* likely to breastfeed; mothers with high scores on AFQT significantly *more* likely to breastfeed; male infants significantly *more* likely to be breastfed; higher birth weight babies significantly *more* likely to be breastfed; African-American babies significantly *less* likely to be breastfed than others; f. relative risk = 1.4491

C.1 a. 2106 cases, 287 drug users; b. CESD mean = 19.72125 for drug users, 15.40462 for nonusers; 76.7% of drug users had gotten high on alcohol, 31.3% of nonusers had gotten high; c. prior probabilities set to existing distribution: .86373 for nonusers, .13628 for users; d. lambda = .8718, $p < .00005$, r_C = .3580, percentage of variance = 12.8 (1.00 − 87.18; $.358^2$); e. D = −1.528810 + 1.840540(ALCOHOL) + .01833649(CESD) + .2019446(DLC); f. ALCOHOL, loading = .88434, all of them; g. 21 women, 8.7%, 86.56%

C.2 a. NSUPPORT, lambda = .87167, F = 77.0358, $p < .00005$; b. ALCOHOL, CESD, DLC, .89786; c. MASTERY, F = .56828, did not enter; d. R_C = .3582, 12.83% of variance; e. the greater the number of social supports, the lower the likelihood of drug use; f. 19 cases, 86.61% correctly classified, negligibly higher percentage than in previous analysis (0.05% higher)

C.3 a. −2 LL = 1399.157, chi-square = 277.841, $p < .00005$; b. 19, 5.9%, 86.28%; c. log [prob (drug use)/prob (no drug use)] = −3.87 + 1.90(ALCOHOL) + .02(CESD) + .34(PROB1) + .11(PROB2) + .35(PROB3) + .01(PROB4) + .02(PROB5) + .26(PROB6) + .52(PROB7) + .12(PROB8) − .02 (PROB9) + .21(PROB10); d. women who got high on alcohol *more* likely to have used drugs; depressed women more likely to have used drugs; women with regular arguments with partner more likely to have used drugs; women with a relative or boyfriend in jail more likely to have used drugs; women with a close friend/relative with a drug or alcohol problem more likely to have used drugs; f. relative risk = 1.6884

CHAPTER 14

A.1 a. recursive; b. endogenous—BMAGEINT and BMAGE1ST; exogenous—BMAGEMEN and BMAFQT80; c. overidentified (no path between V_1 and V_2); d. $z_1 = e_1$, $z_2 = e_2$, $z_3 = p_{31}z_1 + p_{32}z_2 + e_3$, $z_4 = p_{41}z_1 + p_{42}z_2 + p_{43}z_3 + e_4$; e. two

A.2 a. $r_{13} = .092$, $r_{23} = .139$, $r_{14} = .035$, $r_{24} = .352$, $r_{34} = .405$; b. $R = .171$, $R^2 = .029$, $p < .00005$; c. $R = .504$, $R^2 = .254$, $p < .00005$; d. $p_{31} = .09$, $p_{32} = .14$, $p_{41} = .02$, $p_{42} = .30$, $p_{43} = .36$; e. no, p_{41} is not significant ($p = .447$), this path would be trimmed based on statistical criterion *and* on value of $\beta < .05$; f. $e_3 = .985$, $e_4 = .864$

A.3 a. $R = .504$, $R^2 = .254$, $p < .00005$, change $= .00031$; b. $p_{31} = .09$, $p_{32} = .14$, $p_{42} = .30$, $p_{43} = .36$; c. all paths are significant, no theory trimming necessary

C.1 a. exogenous—CESD and NKIDS, endogenous—PSTRESS and HOME@TOT; b. overidentified; c. all are negatively correlated with HOME@TOT; d. the more depressed the mother, the greater parenting stress she perceives; e. two, first regression—dependent = PSTRESS, predictors = NKIDS, CESD, second regression—dependent = HOME@TOT, predictors = NKIDS, CESD, PSTRESS

C.2 a. $R = .339$, $R^2 = .115$, $p < .00005$; b. both are significant at $p < .001$, t (NKIDS) = 3.764, t (CESD) = 15.018; c. $R = .338$, $R^2 = .115$, $p < .00005$; d. $p_{31} = .33$, $p_{32} = .08$, $p_{41} = -.13$, $p_{42} = -.19$, $p_{43} = -.19$; e. yes, none should be trimmed; f. $e_3 = .941$, $e_4 = .941$; g. while all paths are significant, much variance in HOME scores remains to be explained.

C.3 a. no changes—EARNHH is exogenous and is not hypothesized to be related to any other variable in the model; b. $R = .373$, $R^2 = .139$, R^2 change $= .024$; c. $p_{31} = .33$, $p_{32} = .08$, $p_{41} = -.12$, $p_{42} = -.19$, $p_{43} = -.18$, $p_{45} = .16$; d. the explanatory model improved with the inclusion of household earnings; however, as before, much variance in HOME scores remains to be explained.